Stroke Units: An evidence based appr

THE UNIVERSITY C

2

Stroke Units:
An evidence based approach

Peter Langhorne
Senior Lecturer
Academic Section of Geriatric Medicine
Royal Infirmary
Glasgow UK

Martin Dennis
Reader in Stroke Medicine
Neurosciences Trials Unit
University Department of Clinical Neurosciences
Western General Hospital
Edinburgh UK

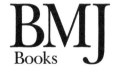

First published in 1998
by BMJ Books, BMA House, Tavistock Square
London WC1H 9JR

British Library Cataloguing in Publication Data

A catalogue record for this book is available from the British Library

ISBN 0-7279-1211-9

Typeset by Apek Typesetters Ltd., Nailsea, Bristol
Printed and bound by Latimer Trend, Plymouth

Contents

Authorship

Peter Langhorne and Martin Dennis have written most chapters and take editorial responsibility for the content and opinions expressed in this book. Additional contributions (Chapter 5 and Appendix) have been made by invited authors. However, many other individuals have contributed to the project and the main body of data, descriptive information, and useful advice and comment have been provided by members of a collaborative review group (the Stroke Unit Trialists' Collaboration – see list below). Therefore individual chapters of the book should be cited as follows: 1, 2, 3, 4, 6 and 7 – Langhorne and Dennis on behalf of the Stroke Unit Trialists' Collaboration; 5 – Major and Walker; Appendix – Perth unit: Hankey and colleagues, Trondheim unit: Indredavik and colleagues, Orpington unit: Kalra, Nottingham unit: Berman and colleagues.

Stroke Unit Trialists' Collaboration (in alphabetical order)

K Asplund, Professor, Umea University Hospital, Umea, Sweden
P Berman, Physician, City Hospital, Nottingham, England
C Blomstrand, Neurologist, Sahlgrenska University Hospital, Goteborg, Sweden
M Dennis, Secretariat: Reader, Western General Hospital, Edinburgh, Scotland
J Douglas, Administrator, University of Glasgow, Scotland
T Erila, Neurologist, Tampere University Hospital, Tampere, Finland
M Garraway, Professor, Public Health Sciences, University of Edinburgh, Scotland
E Hamrin, Professor, Linkoping University, Linkoping, Sweden
G Hankey, Neurologist, Royal Perth Hospital, Perth, Australia
M Ilmavirta, Neurologist, Central Hospital, Jyvaskyla, Finland
B Indredavik, Physician, University Hospital, Trondheim, Norway
L Kalra, Professor, Orpington Hospital, Kent, England
M Kaste, Professor, University of Helsinki, Helsinki, Finland
P Langhorne, Coordinator: Senior Lecturer, Royal Infirmary, Glasgow, Scotland
H Rodgers, Senior Lecturer, University of Newcastle, England
J Sivenius, Professor, University of Kuopio, Kuopio, Finland

J Slattery, Secretariat: Statistician, University of Edinburgh, Scotland

R Stevens, Retired Physician, formerly Dover, England

A Svensson, Professor, Ostra Hospital, Goteborg, Sweden

C Warlow, Secretariat: Professor, Western General Hospital, Edinburgh, Scotland

B Williams, Secretariat: Physician, Gartnavel General Hospital, Glasgow, Scotland

S Wood-Dauphinee, Professor, McGill University, Montreal, Canada

The following people also greatly assisted the project:

D Deleo, Nurse, Royal Perth Hospital, Perth, Australia

A Drummond, Research Fellow, University of Nottingham, England

R Fogelholm, Professor, Central Hospital, Jyvaskyla, Finland

H Palomaki, Neurologist, University of Helsinki, Finland

T Strand, Physician, University Hospital, Umea, Sweden

L Wilhelmsen, Professor, Ostra Hospital, Goteborg, Sweden

Contributors

P Berman, Consultant Physician, Stroke Unit, City Hospital, Nottingham, England.

M Dennis, Reader in Stroke Medicine, Neurosciences Trials Unit, University Department of Clinical Neurosciences, Western General Hospital, Edinburgh, Scotland.

G Hankey, Consultant Neurologist, Stroke Unit, Royal Perth Hospital, Perth, Western Australia.

B Indredavik, Consultant Physician, Stroke Unit, University Hospital, Trondheim, Norway.

L Kalra, Professor and Consultant Physician in Geriatric Medicine, Orpington Hospital, Kent, England.

P Langhorne, Senior Lecturer in Geriatric Medicine, Academic Section of Geriatric Medicine, Royal Infirmary, Glasgow, Scotland.

K Major, Health Economist, Ayrshire and Arran Health Board, Boswell House, Ayr, Scotland.

A Walker, Health Economist, Greater Glasgow Health Board, Ingram Street, Glasgow, Scotland.

Foreword

It is now several years since I gave up being a researcher and more than two decades since I left clinical practice in the more capable hands of others. This has made it increasingly easy for me to view research from the perspective of a potential patient. It is from that perspective, and from the perspective of an occasional carer of relatives who have experienced strokes, that I suggest that the work described in this book is of immense importance. As Peter Langhorne and Martin Dennis note in their Preface, there has been controversy for over three decades about whether an improvement in the organisation of care for stroke patients can help them to remain independent. Some high quality evaluative studies have been done over that period, but it was only very recently that anyone had identified and then reviewed them using methods likely to reduce biases and the play of chance. Once prepared, a systematic review of the evidence from controlled trials made clear that there was very strong support for the views of those who had maintained that proper organisation of stroke care could be expected to improve patients' chances of recovery. Of particular importance for those of us who fear survival with a severe disability even more than death, the review showed that organised stroke care increased not only the likelihood of survival but also the likelihood of avoiding subsequent institutionalisation.

The importance of this discovery – for that is what has been achieved by the Stroke Unit Trialists' Collaboration – can hardly be over-emphasised. When the Cochrane Database of Systematic Reviews was launched by the Minister for Health in London on 24 April 1995, it was the Cochrane review of stroke units which was selected to illustrate the potential power of discoveries based on careful analyses of existing research evidence. The challenge now is to ensure that patients who can benefit from organised stroke care actually receive it. One of the ways to promote this objective is to ensure that the public becomes familiar with the strength of evidence presented in this book. In this way, members of the public and those representing their interests will be well equipped to lobby, where necessary, for better services for stroke patients. What are the lessons from the experience described in this book? One is that patients would have been better served if the spirit of co-operative research exemplified by the Stroke Unit Trialists' Collaboration had existed throughout the three decades over which debate has existed about the value of organising stroke care properly. Stroke researchers and funding agencies owe it to future patients to build on the collaboration which has led to the discoveries presented in this book. Furthermore, if they invite past and future stroke patients to help them to develop their plans for future research, I predict that they are likely to make relevant discoveries far more rapidly in future than they have done in the past. Indeed, if they are looking for volunteers for future, well designed, collaborative trials, I offer myself as a potential participant – particularly one comparing organised domiciliary care with organised hospital care!

Iain Chalmers
UK Cochrane Centre

Preface

What is the most effective way to provide care for stroke patients admitted to hospital? The question is important because stroke is a condition which is common, often fatal or disabling, and expensive[1] and traditional approaches to providing stroke care have been widely criticised as being haphazard and lacking evidence of benefit.[2] A central issue has been whether an improvement in the organisation of care for stroke patients (the stroke unit model of care) can produce worthwhile, tangible benefits for the patients who receive that care. This question has been surprisingly controversial for over 30 years despite being specifically addressed by several high quality research studies.

In this book we explore the reasons why the stroke unit model of care has been seen as controversial and then readdress the question of how best to organise stroke care using the best evidence available from randomised clinical trials. Finally, we use this information to try to guide the planning and delivery of inpatient stroke care. We have provided introductory information on clinical trials and systematic reviews on the assumption that many readers will not have prior knowledge. We hope this book will be of interest to members of all professions who wish to develop evidence based practices in providing care for stroke patients. Unfortunately this book, like most books, will rapidly become outdated as more research evidence becomes available. Those who wish to keep up to date with new developments will find updated versions of the stroke unit systematic review in the Cochrane Library.[3]

We are most grateful to Carl Counsell and Hazel Fraser of the Cochrane Collaboration Stroke Group for invaluable assistance with literature searching, Iain Chalmers for advice on the manuscript, Patricia McCusker for secretarial support, Chest Heart and Stroke Scotland for financial support of the Stroke Unit Trialists' Collaboration project, and our families who have tolerated yet another intrusion into their lives.

Peter Langhorne
Martin Dennis

1: The stroke unit story

There is a long history of research examining whether organised (stroke unit) care improves the recovery of stroke patients in hospital. Despite this research, as recently as 1992 there was no clear consensus about the benefit of this form of care. Two major factors may explain this:

1. many research studies were of a design which could not provide reliable answers;
2. no systematic evaluation of the available research had been performed.

In this book we set out to describe such an evaluation and draw practical lessons from it, for both health care and research.

History of stroke unit care and its evaluation

Stroke is both common and serious. It has been estimated that in 1990 stroke caused 4.4 million deaths worldwide.[1] Within most Western countries a typical district of 250,000 people might expect more than 500 new strokes per year,[2] of whom a half will have died or remain physically dependent one year later.[3] Because so many survivors remain disabled, stroke related disability is common and its prevalence has been estimated at over 6/1000 in the general population.[4] In addition to its impact on the health of the population, stroke also imposes a huge cost on health services. Almost 5% of all health service costs in the UK[5] and over 3% of the Dutch annual health care budget[6] is attributed to stroke care. In the UK, stroke accounts for almost 6% of all hospital costs and figures from other Western countries are likely to be at least as great.[7] Furthermore, since the costs of caring for disabled survivors are likely to dominate the lifetime costs of stroke,[6] the financial burden to society as a whole is likely to be huge.

Although many would argue that the research efforts directed at optimising the management of stroke have been disproportionately small given its enormous personal, social, and financial costs, many studies over the last 50 years have attempted to evaluate different models of stroke care. In this chapter we will attempt to trace the development of stroke units. This account is inevitably based on

1

published reports and takes no account of unreported efforts to introduce novel stroke services.

Early studies

Some of the first studies of the organisation of stroke care came from Northern Ireland[8] during the 1950s (Box 1.1). Adams[8] reported experiences from the establishment of a stroke rehabilitation unit within a department of geriatric medicine which indicated that the proportion of patients regaining sufficient functional independence to return home was increased after the development of this new service. They also observed a reduction in the number of patients who died within the first two months of their stroke. During the 1960s further small observational studies (see [9–11]) suggested that organised stroke care, focused around a stroke rehabilitation team based within a stroke unit, could result in improvements in the recovery of stroke patients. Unfortunately, none of these results were convincing because they were based on observational studies which compared the new service with

---

Box 1.1   "Landmarks" in the history of stroke unit care

1950   First published reports of organised stroke care[8]
1962   First published RCT of a system of stroke rehabilitation[34]
1970   Reports (no (RCTs) of stroke intensive care units[19]
1970s   Early definitions and descriptions of a "stroke unit"[12,17]
1980   First large (> 300 patients) RCT of a stroke unit shows only short term benefits[22]
1985   RCT of a mobile stroke team[27]
1988   King's Fund Consensus Conference statement criticises stroke services[30]
1990   Small systematic review suggests possible benefits of stroke unit care[16]
1991   RCT of a stroke unit provides convincing evidence of benefit[35]
1993   First RCT of an acute stroke unit (intervening only in the first few days)[36]
1993   Systematic review (ten RCTs) suggests stroke unit care may prevent premature deaths[37]
1995   Pan European Consensus Meeting supports organised stroke unit care[38]
1997   Updated systematic review (18 RCTs) shows a reduction in dependency[14]

RCT, randomised controlled trial

---

previous experience (historical controls). The reasons why this is an unreliable source of information are explained below (Levels of evidence, Chapter 2).

Definitions of a stroke unit

During these early investigations into the organisation of stroke care a number of the principles and components of stroke unit care became established and the first definitions of a "stroke unit" were published. Stroke units were variously defined as:

- a team of specialists who are knowledgeable about the care of the stroke patient and who consult throughout a hospital wherever a patient may be;[12]
- a special area of a hospital that provides beds for stroke patients who are cared for by a team of specialists;[13]
- a geographic location within the hospital designated for stroke and stroke-like patients who are in need of rehabilitation services and skilled professional care that such a unit can provide.[14]

In each case stroke units were seen as providing focused care for stroke patients comprising elements of specialism and organisation.

These early studies also established that most stroke units were staffed by a core multidisciplinary team which would usually comprise medical, nursing, therapy, and social work staff (Box 1.2). Some early stroke units[15] also involved other disciplines such as dieticians, neurologists, ophthalmologists, chaplains, neuro-psychologists, and audiologists. It also became recognised[16] that these multidisciplinary groups developed co-ordinated policies and procedures to formulate and execute an integrated rehabilitation plan tailored to the individual patient's problems and needs (Box 1.3). The main advantage of having specialised units for stroke

---

Box 1.2 Disciplines represented in the "core" multidisciplinary team

Medical
Nursing
Physiotherapy
Occupational therapy
Speech and language therapy
Social work

Box 1.3   Principles of stroke unit care

Comprehensive assessment of all aspects of the patient's illness and disability

Close collaboration between the disciplines involved

Identification and awareness of the objectives of rehabilitation

A role in education and research on stroke disease

---

patients was said to be that it provided the opportunity to develop these collaborative policies for stroke rehabilitation.[17]

Stroke intensive care units

During these early years of developing stroke rehabilitation units an alternative movement, mainly based in the United States, was setting up and evaluating intensive care units for stroke patients. These stroke intensive care units were comparable to coronary care units but unlike them, they never became widely established.[18] The original rationale was that a high intensity nursing input, specialist medical investigations, close monitoring, and standardised procedures for diagnosis, investigation, and management would reduce early stroke mortality. The first published evaluation of intensive care for stroke compared the outcome of patients admitted to a newly established "acute neurovascular intensive care unit" with those treated in two community hospitals.[19] Although the study design could not ensure that comparable patients were allocated to the two types of service, the study groups were reasonably similar with respect to certain key prognostic variables.[19] This study failed to show any impact of the "acute neurovascular unit" on mortality and morbidity, but there did appear to be a reduction in post-stroke complications. Other similar studies published around the same time[20,21] also failed to show any convincing benefit from this type of stroke unit. However, none of these studies used appropriate methods or was of sufficient size reliably to demonstrate whether these models of care were or were not effective (Levels of evidence, Chapter 2).

Later developments

With the declining interest in stroke intensive care units, new approaches were developed in the 1970s and 1980s. In particular, researchers experimented with models of care where stroke patients were recruited early after their stroke but could receive a prolonged period of rehabilitation if necessary (i.e. combined acute and rehabilitation care, sometimes referred to as "acute rehabilitation units"). Published examples appeared from North America,[14,15] Britain[22] and Scandinavia.[23,24] The rationale for these units was that stroke patients should receive the bulk of their care within a specialist area, acknowledging the principles that rehabilitation in its broadest sense should start very early and that continuity of care is important.

During this period there were also some reports of stroke rehabilitation units where patients were admitted after an initial delay of one or two weeks after stroke onset (for example[17,25,26]). Broadly speaking, the philosophy of care in these services was similar to that in "acute rehabilitation units" although this model inevitably introduced a delay in applying these rehabilitation principles and reduced continuity of care. Mobile stroke teams, which attempted to bring co-ordinated multidisciplinary care to patients housed in a variety of non-specialist wards,[27,28] were also described and evaluated in the 1980s. Some quite detailed descriptions of practice also appeared (for example[17,29]) outlining the units' operational policies. Many of these stroke units admitted only selected patients, the prevailing view being that patients in the "middle band" of stroke severity would derive most benefit from stroke unit care.[13,14] During this period researchers also began to use more rigorous methods, including randomised trials, to evaluate stroke units (Box 1.1) which probably reflected the increasing awareness of the strengths and weaknesses of different methods of treatment evaluation within medicine in general. Prior to 1980, most studies had simply described the experience of a stroke unit and compared its results with another hospital or with historical controls.

By the end of the 1980s, there appeared to be some consensus (Box 1.4) based on the results of several small randomised trials that stroke unit care may speed up recovery after stroke but that

---

Box 1.4   Conventional interpretation of stroke unit trials

The conventional view in 1990 was that stroke units:

- may speed up recovery after stroke
- have no influence on survival
- have no influence on long term functional outcomes

5

survival or long term recovery were unlikely to be improved.[4,16] Around this time, Garraway[13] identified several other unresolved issues regarding stroke unit practice which included the appropriate selection of patients, the appropriate mix of resources within stroke units, the ideal size of a stroke unit, and the optimal method of providing continuing management after discharge from the unit.

The uncertainty about the value of stroke units probably contributed to the findings of the King's Fund Consensus Panel in 1988[30] that stroke services in the UK were generally haphazard and poorly tailored to the patients' needs. As recently as 1993, a national postal survey of all UK hospital consultants who cared for stroke showed that less than half had access to specialised stroke rehabilitation units.[31] In contrast, Scandinavian countries such as Norway (Indredavik, personal communication) and Sweden[32] were moving toward more uniform provision of stroke unit care.

The demands of evidence based practice

Evidence based medicine,[33] the explicit linking of clinical practice to the most reliable clinical research evidence, has been seen as one of the major recent developments in the practice and evaluation of health care. It is interesting to re-examine the evolution of stroke units from this perspective. Stroke units were initially established on the premise that they would offer a better system of care by bringing together the many skills and disciplines required to provide comprehensive management of the multitude of problems a stroke patient may experience. However, critics argued (quite reasonably) that if we intend to reorganise services and possibly increase expenditure, we should have evidence that such reorganisation will bring about worthwhile benefits for patients and for the health service in general. As we have already seen, many research studies were carried out to examine the potential benefits of stroke unit care. However, despite three decades of discussion and research, by 1990 there was still no clear consensus about the value of stroke units. This uncertainty resulted from our failure either to systematically review the results of the available research or to perform really large, methodologically robust randomised trials. Either of these approaches could have provided much more reliable evidence of the effectiveness (or otherwise) of stroke unit care.

In this book we will describe a systematic review of the relevant research studies which has examined the question of whether stroke unit care can improve patient outcomes compared with alternative systems of care. To do this, we must first consider some of the methodological problems which arise when evaluating health care interventions (treatments) and in particular when evaluating complex health service interventions. Having described the results of our review, we will discuss their implications for the organisation of stroke care in hospital.

2: How should we evaluate our interventions?

When examining the evidence for health service interventions, we should place most emphasis on those research studies which provide the most reliable results: randomised controlled trials. However, even high quality research trials may individually be too small or too locally specific to answer our questions reliably. Systematic reviews, despite having their own problems and limitations, can provide a useful synthesis of evidence from several primary trials.

Levels of evidence

The primary aim of health services research is to provide reliable information on how to organise services to bring about the greatest benefit for patients. Therefore we must give most emphasis to research methods which can produce reliable results. When considering the evidence for or against the effectiveness of a particular intervention (treatment or service) it is widely accepted that certain types of evidence are more reliable than others for guiding clinical practice.[1] These criteria are summarised in Table 2.1. The least reliable approach (level IV) is to base clinical practice only on one's own or somebody else's experience, especially where that is based on memory (i.e. anecdotal evidence). We are likely to place most emphasis on our most recent, most successful or most unsuccessful experiences.[1]

A systematic collection of information on a series of patients (uncontrolled case series) can overcome the problems of selective memory (level III). However, in a condition like stroke where the outcome for an individual patient is so difficult to predict, it is usually impossible to conclude that a particular intervention is superior to another unless the difference in effectiveness is very large.[1] This problem can be circumvented by comparing the outcomes of patients treated in a particular way with others (controls) treated using an alternative strategy. One can use

Table 2.1   Types of evidence about health care interventions

Level	Type of evidence
Ia	Evidence obtained from a meta-analysis of randomised controlled trials
Ib	Evidence obtained from at least one randomised controlled trial
IIa	Evidence obtained from at least one well designed controlled study without randomisation
IIb	Evidence obtained from at least one other type of well designed experimental study
III	Evidence obtained from well designed non-experimental descriptive studies, such as comparative studies, correlation studies, and case studies
IV	Evidence obtained from expert committee reports or opinions and/or experiences of respected authorities

Based on guidelines published by the US Department and Human Services Agency for Health Care Policy and Research.[1]

historical controls where the outcomes of patients treated in a novel way are compared with those previously treated using a traditional approach. Unfortunately, significant differences in outcome can occur which are nothing to do with the intervention under investigation. Over time, systematic differences may develop in the types of patients (for example, severity of disease), in the general management of the patients (other services and treatments available), and in the methods of measuring their outcomes.[2] To avoid this possibility, a contemporary control group (concurrent controls) should be identified at the same time as the treatment group (level II). However, even where one identifies a concurrent control group, two major sources of error remain:[3] systematic error (also termed "bias") and random error (Box 2.1). Fortunately both of these can be overcome by large randomised controlled trials (i.e. level I).

Box 2.1   Sources of error in studies of health care interventions

1. Systematic error (bias)
   - (i)   Selection bias
   - (ii) Performance bias
   - (iii) Attrition bias
   - (iv) Recording bias
2. Random error

Sources of error

Systematic error (bias)

Bias occurs when the design of the research study produces a systematic distortion of the results away from the "true" value. Therefore, sources of bias can influence the validity of a trial, i.e. the degree to which the trial result approximates to the truth (also termed the "internal validity" of a study – the degree to which the results are likely to be true for the patient group studied). There are many potential sources of bias, some of which can be controlled or prevented through careful design of the research study.[3] Figure 2.1 outlines some of the main sources of bias in a study which compares a new treatment (termed "intervention") with the normal care available (termed "control"). The potential sources of bias are as follows.

Selection bias (systematic pretreatment differences in comparison groups)

This is probably the main source of bias in health services research and is the reason why randomised controlled trials are regarded as the "gold standard".[4] In a randomised trial a random process (for example, a computerised randomisation system)

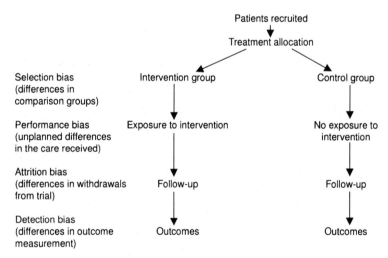

Figure 2.1   Sources of bias in research trials. This outlines the four main sources of bias identified in clinical research trials. (Adapted from the Cochrane Handbook.[3])

determines whether a patient receives the intervention or the control service and so the two patient groups should (by random chance) have very similar characteristics. Any non-random way of assigning patients to comparison groups, for example using home address, patient preference, professional preference, will often produce systematic differences between the two patient groups such that one group will stand a better chance of doing well regardless of the care they receive. For example, if the effects of a health promotion programme were examined by comparing the health of individuals who chose to take part as opposed to those who chose not to do so, then people who were interested in their health would inevitably end up in the health promotion group. As these people were more likely to enjoy good health anyway, the study would probably suggest a positive benefit from health promotion regardless of whether the programme really was effective. Statistical techniques exist which help correct for differences between two study groups but these are imperfect and can only correct for differences which we know about and can measure. Randomisation avoids biases from factors which we do not know about and cannot measure.

It is important to appreciate that even good randomisation procedures can produce unequal study groups if based on small numbers of patients. This is due to random chance (see Random error, below) and can only really be avoided by recruiting sufficiently large numbers of patients.

Performance bias (systematic differences in the care provided apart from the intervention being evaluated)

Performance bias simply acknowledges that if we wish to study a particular intervention then all other aspects of a patient's care should be similar in the intervention and control groups. Where a double blind trial design is used (i.e. neither the patient nor those caring for them know whether the patient is in the treatment or control group – easily achieved in placebo controlled drug trials), the patients in each group should by chance receive very similar general (non-trial) care. This is relatively easy to achieve in drug trials but difficult to achieve in complex health service or rehabilitation trials. Where blinding is inadequate, ineffective or simply not possible because of the nature of the intervention, systematic differences may develop in the general (non-trial) care the treatment and control patients receive. For example, in an open (unblinded) trial of a particularly hazardous drug such as streptokinase in ischaemic stroke, the staff may more carefully monitor those patients known to have received the drug. Any observed improvement in outcomes may reflect the more intensive monitoring and careful general care rather than the drug itself.

Attrition bias (systematic differences in withdrawals from the trials)

To obtain a reliable result from a trial it is essential to follow up all the patients who joined the study because patients who are withdrawn from or stop participating in a study tend to differ from those who remain in the study. A simple example would be a rehabilitation trial where the main outcome was a disability score (for example, the Barthel index). In this hypothetical example, the control group patients who had severe strokes did badly and were more likely to die or withdraw from the study because of medical complications. However, at the end of the trial the control group appeared to have done better than the intervention group because the Barthel Index of those patients who remained was higher (i.e. the attrition had removed from the final analysis those ill patients who had severe strokes and would have had a low Barthel index). This type of bias is avoided by performing an "intention to treat analysis" where the analysis of results at the end of the study includes every patient who was assigned (allocated) to the intervention or control group, regardless of whether they subsequently dropped out of the trial.

Detection bias (systematic differences in outcome assessment)

Detection bias is a major problem in rehabilitation research where the outcomes (e.g. disability score) are measured by an assessor. If the assessor has any (either conscious or unconscious) notion about which treatment is more effective then there is a real danger that this will influence the way in which they assess the health of patients in the two study groups. The problem is less marked with objective outcomes such as death or survival. The best method for limiting this form of bias is to carry out a "blinded" assessment of a patient's outcome where the researcher carrying out the assessment is unaware of the treatment the patient received. There is now empirical evidence from rehabilitation research[5] that studies with a blinded assessment of outcome produce more modest estimates of the effectiveness of interventions than studies where the assessor was aware of which patients received the intervention.

Random error

It is a fact of life that measurements of any natural system tend to vary in a random way around some average or "true" value. The larger the number of participants studied, the smaller this imprecision (error) will become. For example, if one wishes to know the average blood pressure of patients who have suffered a stroke, a sample of ten patients will produce an imprecise estimate whereas a sample of 1000 is likely to provide a very close approximation to the "true" value. This is an important concept in controlled trials where we usually judge the effectiveness of an intervention by comparing estimates of the "average" outcome in the intervention group with the "average" outcome in the controls.

Design of a reliable stroke unit trial

To determine reliably whether a stroke unit improves patient outcomes, our ideal research study would have several features. It would ensure that:

- sufficient numbers of patients are recruited to ensure sufficient statistical power to overcome the effects of random error;
- patients are randomly allocated to the novel (stroke unit) intervention or the conventional care (control) service in a way which produces a very similar mix of patients in each group;
- patients in the stroke unit do not receive (or avoid) any additional treatments other than those which are part of the stroke unit "package";
- all patients who are allocated to the stroke unit or conventional care are followed up until the end of the study and that the final analysis is based on the group to which they were originally allocated;
- the outcomes used at the end of the study are recorded in such a way to reduce the risk of bias.

Clinical trials are only useful if they provide information which is relevant as well as reliable. Therefore the information obtained must be of interest to all who wish to use the trial results to make treatment choices (patients, carers, purchasers, providers) and should include costs and satisfaction with care as well as the more conventional death and disability outcomes.

Why randomised trials may not be enough

We have outlined the main reasons why well designed randomised trials are likely to provide the least biased and hence most reliable evaluation of whether stroke unit care is effective. However, even very rigorous and carefully conducted randomised trials are unlikely on their own to provide all the information we require. There are two main reasons for this.

Sample size

Most individual hospitals would not admit enough stroke patients over a two or three year period to support a randomised trial of sufficient size to reduce random error and reliably answer all the questions of interest. In fact, one of the main reasons why no clear consensus had developed around the existing stroke unit trials is probably that none of these individual studies were of sufficient size to produce a convincing, reliable result. One can calculate[6] that a stroke unit trial designed to reliably detect a modest reduction in the number of patients who die would need to recruit thousands of patients whereas the largest trial recruited barely over 400 patients. For example, for a trial to reliably detect a result where 20% of patients die in the stroke unit group compared with 25% of the controls – which represents a 5% absolute reduction (i.e. 25–20%) and 20% relative reduction (i.e. 5% divided by 25%) in deaths – would require 2000 patients.

Generalisability

Trials carried out in a single hospital will inevitably test a system of care operating within local circumstances. Therefore, even if a stroke unit was shown to be effective in one hospital, we may be uncertain whether a similar system of care would be effective if established in another centre. We could argue that other factors might be important; for example, the staff working in the stroke unit may have been particularly skilled or the conventional services may have been particularly poor. Even well conducted trials (with good internal validity) may not tell us about the best care for the types of patients who were not entered into the trial. This aspect of a trial is termed its "external validity" and reflects the degree to which the trial results are generalisable (applicable) elsewhere. Trials of relatively simple interventions (for example, aspirin[7,8]) are easier to generalise than those of more complex surgical interventions (for example, carotid surgery[9]). Rehabilitation and service interventions provide us with the greatest challenges.

14

One way to avoid these problems which has been used extensively in drug research is to carry out a multicentre trial. In these trials the number of patients recruited is greatly increased by planning a simple trial which can be carried out on multiple sites, often in multiple countries. Not only does this provide greater patient numbers but it gives increased confidence that the treatment can work in many different settings. The particular advantages of multicentre trials over reviews of several smaller trials are that patient selection, randomisation, the definition and delivery of interventions, and recording of outcomes can all be standardised.

Unfortunately, multicentre trials are very difficult to organise for rehabilitation interventions[10] which tend to be very expensive and complex. It is impossible to replicate exactly the treatment in different centres as there will always be some local differences in the services available. For these reasons multicentre trials of rehabilitation interventions have been uncommon (although attempts have been made, for example in cardiac rehabilitation[11,12] and occupational therapy after stroke (Gladman, personal communication)). An alternative (and complementary) approach is to make the best use of the available randomised trials by carrying out a systematic review.

Systematic reviews of randomised trials

Conduct of systematic reviews

If large randomised trials are impractical, we have to draw the most reliable conclusions from smaller trials. Unfortunately, the conventional approach, the narrative review, is unreliable.[13] Conventional reviews usually fail to define the review question, to ensure that all relevant trials are reviewed and assessed in an unbiased manner, or to draw conclusions which are explicitly based on the evidence. Systematic reviews set out to improve upon narrative reviews by applying scientific methods to the review of research evidence.[14] They synthesise the results of multiple primary investigations (trials) using strategies that limit both random error and systematic error (bias). These strategies[3] include:

- defining the *research question* to ensure the review will be relevant and reliable and to guide the development of the review protocol. A major decision is how broad to make the question; too narrow a question may identify too few trials and reduce statistical

15

power, while too broad a question may waste effort and result in a systematic review which is difficult to interpret. A compromise approach (e.g. Antiplatelet Trialists' Collaboration[15]) is to begin with a broad question (Do antiplatelet drugs prevent vascular disease?) which includes specified subquestions (e.g. Does low dose aspirin prevent recurrent stroke in the elderly?);

- developing a review *protocol* based on the research question to reduce the risk of bias in trial selection by specifying the criteria by which trials will be included or excluded from the review;
- conducting a *comprehensive search* for all potentially relevant information to ensure that all relevant trials are identified and included in the review;
- *selecting trials* using prespecified, explicit and reproducible methods to reduce the risk of bias in trial selection;
- performing a *critical appraisal* of the characteristics and research designs of the primary studies to ensure that most emphasis is given to the most reliable trials;
- using explicit methods of *data extraction and synthesis* to minimise bias during data collection and the analysis of results;
- *interpreting* the findings in a way which is clearly linked to all the available evidence.

A statistical synthesis (meta-analysis) of the results is often undertaken at the end of such a process (see What is meta-analysis?, p 33 Chapter 4) but systematic reviews can be carried out without any formal statistical analysis being performed.[3]

Thus systematic reviews provide a method of reviewing the available evidence using explicit scientific strategies to minimise the risk of bias. They should provide the least biased summary of the available research evidence and may provide invaluable pointers to future research and the best estimate of the effects (effectiveness) of a particular treatment (Box 2.2). However, systematic reviews also have their problems and limitations which can arise from problems of bias (systematic error) or interpretation.

Box 2.2 Potential role of systematic reviews

1. Provide most reliable summary of available information
2. Provide invaluable pointers to future research
3. *May* provide best estimate of whether a particular treatment is effective

---

Sources of bias in systematic reviews

Sources of bias in systematic reviews are important as they may make the results of the review unreliable. They can be subdivided as follows.

Publication bias

One of the central methods for reducing bias in systematic reviews is to ensure that all the relevant trials are identified and included. Unfortunately, not only is this difficult but those studies which are easy to find tend to differ from those which are difficult to find. The reason for this is that research studies which have produced an interesting (and usually "positive" result) are more likely to be published than those which produce an unexciting or neutral result.[16,17] This phenomenon is known as "publication bias". We can try to circumvent this by using multiple sources of information when searching for trials (electronic databases such as Medline and Embase include only a certain number of journals within a limited range of languages) and to actively seek information on theses, conference abstracts, and unpublished trials.

Study quality bias

Systematic reviews can only be as good as the primary research studies they include. There is good empirical evidence[18] that trials which have used less reliable methods tend to indicate that new treatments are more effective than do the more methodologically robust trials. In dealing with this problem, it is important to establish the methodological quality of the studies included within the systematic review (in particular those characteristics which are designed to reduce bias – Figure 2.1) and to interpret the review accordingly.

Outcome recording bias

It is important that the relevant outcomes are recorded in a similar way within different trials. Problems may arise where individual trials have published their most impressive results and not reported their least impressive results. There is then a danger that if all the published results are combined, one will simply be "cherry-picking" the most interesting results from each study.[19] This problem can be minimised by deciding in advance which outcomes are to be used and collecting the data in a consistent way from each study.

Interpretation of systematic reviews

The second area of difficulty with systematic reviews concerns their interpretation. The simplest form of systematic review is one which has examined a relatively simple treatment (for example, a drug) which has been tested in a number of randomised controlled trials within a narrow dose range and in relatively similar groups of patients. In practice, this scenario is uncommon and diversity can occur at several levels within the primary randomised trials.[3] These areas of diversity can be categorised as follows.

Participants

Different randomised trials may recruit different types of participants (patients). This could influence the results of the trial if the particular intervention is only effective within one particular group of patients. For this reason it is important to know something about the characteristics of the patients recruited into the original (primary) trials.

Context

Different randomised trials are carried out within the context of different background health care services. For instance, a randomised trial of a new rehabilitation service established in the United States would have a very different context (and hence control services) than if it was established in the United Kingdom.

Methods

We have outlined in Systematic error (bias) (p 10) the reasons why randomised controlled trials are regarded as the "gold standard" for evaluating new treatments. However, randomised trials can be carried out with greater or lesser degrees of rigour. Undue emphasis on the less rigorous trials will increase the risk of introducing bias.[18]

Interventions

A major challenge with stroke rehabilitation studies is that the intervention itself is likely to be very complex and non-uniform. Any intervention delivered by a therapist or a multidisciplinary team will involve many components which may interact in different ways. It is likely that these interventions may include a mixture of both effective and ineffective elements so it is important that we are aware of the variability between the different trials and that we explore this variability when analysing the results.

Certain safeguards can be built into the conduct of a systematic review. Firstly, we must be aware of where there may be variation between the characteristics of the primary studies (this is termed "heterogeneity"[3]). This can include the characteristics of patients recruited, the setting of the trial, the trial methods, and the interventions. Secondly, we should explore the influence of this heterogeneity on the results of the systematic review.[20] This can be done through "subgroup" or "sensitivity" analyses where the results of a systematic review are re-analysed excluding trials which exhibit particular characteristics. In this way we can examine to what degree our conclusions depend on trials with particular characteristics (NB: there are methodological limitations to this process which are outlined in Subgroup analysis, p46 Chapter 4). Finally, we must interpret the results of these analyses with caution to provide an honest account of how certain we can be about the conclusions.

3:   Assembling evidence about stroke units

This systematic review was based on a broad review question identifying 19 relevant randomised trials of organised (stroke unit) care. Descriptive information from these trials indicated consistent differences between the organised (stroke unit) care and conventional care. These were: the presence of co-ordinated multidisciplinary team care, specialist interests of the staff in stroke and/or rehabilitation, the involvement of carers in the rehabilitation process, and the provision of programmes of education and training in stroke.

Formulating the stroke unit question

We indicated in Chapter 2 that most systematic reviews begin with a question which is used to develop a protocol incorporating the trial inclusion and exclusion criteria, the search strategy, and the methods of data analysis.[1] One of the first decisions is how broad the review question should be; too broad may waste effort and create difficulties of interpretation, too narrow may result in too few trials being identified. However, it is often possible to ask a broad general question which incorporates several narrower subquestions.

Defining the intervention

We have a number of pieces of information from the stroke unit literature which could guide the formulation of our broad question (see Chapter 1, p 3–4). Firstly, we knew that although the various historical definitions of "stroke unit" incorporated a variety of features (for example, a specialist stroke ward, a multidisciplinary team of specialists, a specialist with an interest in rehabilitation, and the co-ordination of care within specialist units), the definitions all incorporated two key features:

1. they were hospital based;
2. they incorporated some attempt to improve the organisation of care.

Secondly, even if stroke units were believed to be effective there was continuing uncertainty around other more specific questions:[2]

- What type of stroke unit is effective? To answer this, we wished to include trials of different types of unit. For example, a disease-specific stroke ward or mobile stroke team or services where there was an attempt to improve the organisation of stroke care within a generic disability service (i.e. services also catering for disabling illnesses other than stroke);
- What are the important components and practices within a stroke unit? It seemed likely that many of the trials would have evaluated a unit which met a specific stroke unit definition[3] such as "multidisciplinary team of specialist staff serving as a focus for clinical care, teaching and research". However, we did not wish to define our intervention so specifically at this early stage but to "cast a net broadly" to catch all those systems of organised inpatient stroke care which had been evaluated in randomised trials.

Therefore, we used the term "stroke unit" to refer to a system of organisation of care rather than necessarily a physical ward.

Defining the patient group

The next part of our question concerned the patient group which would be studied. It seemed sensible to set our criteria as broadly as possible to ensure that the systematic review included the maximum number of relevant trials. We expected that most studies would have recruited acute stroke patients and used a clinical definition of stroke since many of the trials predated computerised tomography scanning. We would therefore expect them to have included both ischaemic and haemorrhagic strokes which met the World Health Organisation clinical definition (paraphrased as "a focal neurological deficit caused by vascular disease"[4]). In most countries subarachnoid haemorrhage is managed in a substantially different manner to other strokes (often involving neurosurgery) and so these would routinely be excluded from stroke unit studies. We could therefore define our stroke patient group as those having recently suffered an illness which met an accepted clinical definition of stroke.

Previous authors[2] have raised the question of which patient groups might benefit from stroke unit care. In particular, it was suggested that patients in a "middle band" of stroke severity (excluding very mild and very severe strokes) would gain the most benefit. Therefore information on stroke severity was sought as a possible factor which might influence the effectiveness of stroke unit care.

Defining the context

It seemed likely that within the randomised trials stroke unit care would have been compared with different types of control service. The most pragmatic approach was therefore to include any trial which compared stroke unit care with the contemporary conventional care but to subdivide the latter into different groups (for example, general medical ward, geriatric medical assessment unit).

Defining the outcomes

When deciding which outcomes to focus upon, it is useful to think of all the outcomes likely to be meaningful to those people, including patients, who will make health care decisions on the basis of the systematic review.[1] We therefore considered outcomes such as death, disability, the requirement for institutional care, the length of stay in a hospital or institution, satisfaction with services, and quality of life.

Using this background information, we formulated a broad question to guide the systematic review: "Can stroke unit care improve the outcomes of stroke patients?" (Figure 3.1). Within this broad question we could define a stroke unit trial as one which has focused on inpatient (within hospital) care where an attempt was

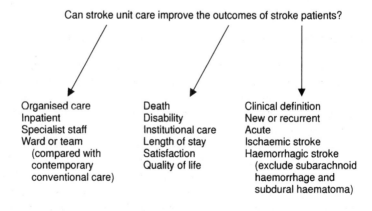

Figure 3.1 Broad question for the systematic review.

made to improve the organisation of stroke care compared with the contemporary conventional care.

Identifying the relevant trials

One of the distinguishing characteristics of a systematic review is the use of a comprehensive unbiased search for the available evidence (Conduct of systematic reviews, Chapter 2). We were fortunate in having the support of the Cochrane Collaboration Stroke Review Group[5] whose efforts were supplemented by additional search strategies. In summary, our approach included the following:

- systematic handsearching of 22 core neurology and stroke journals;
- systematic handsearches of five Japanese journals;
- systematic searches of Medline and Embase;
- searching of the reference lists of trials, review articles and textbooks relevant to stroke care;
- searching of *Current Contents* plus the proceedings of 43 recent conferences in neurology, geriatric medicine, and rehabilitation;
- systematic searches of dissertation abstracts;
- conversation and correspondence with colleagues in the area of stroke care;
- publicising preliminary findings at stroke conferences in the United Kingdom, Scandinavia, Germany, Switzerland, Spain, Canada, and South America.

Locating information from relevant trials

It is important that data are collected from relevant trials in a manner which is reproducible and which will minimise bias (Conduct of systematic reviews, Chapter 2). Therefore we invited the principal investigators of each trial which fulfilled our inclusion criteria to join a collaborative group (Stroke Unit Trialists' Collaboration[6]). This approach has been shown to facilitate the collection of more detailed information about individual trials.[7] All who could be contacted agreed to join. They were then asked to provide details of their trial design, including descriptive information about the stroke unit intervention and the conventional care. This was carried out through a structured interview with each trial co-ordinator and was supplemented with other sources of information, including a questionnaire. This focused on aspects of the structure, staffing, organisation, selection criteria, and the procedures and practices within the stroke unit and conventional care settings.

The stroke unit trials

General comments

Using our broad selection criteria, we identified 19 randomised trials which compared a more organised system of inpatient (stroke unit) care with the less organised conventional care. Although the two researchers who had independently assessed the trials showed good agreement in deciding which trials fulfilled the systematic review inclusion criteria, we were still faced with the problem of comparing two ill defined systems of care. We therefore examined some of the basic components within the stroke unit and conventional care settings to ensure that our broad definition had identified the interventions and control services which we were interested in studying. If these components were consistent within the different types of stroke unit care then we could be more confident that we were reviewing the relevant trials. We also wished to know if the stroke units differed from each other in the methods used (for example, method of randomisation, blinding of follow-up; Systematic error bias, Chapter 2). We therefore defined, at the start of the systematic review, a number of different categories of stroke care (Box 3.1).

Stroke unit characteristics

Of the 19 trials our search and selection process had identified, 17 ([8-23]; Svensson et al, unpublished data) had used formal randomisation procedures and a further two[24,25] used a less rigorous system of treatment allocation (quasi-random; treatment allocated by bed availability or day of hospital admission). These two trials were evaluated separately to exclude significant bias in our conclusions. An outline of the design of all these trials is provided in Table 3.1. The organised (stroke unit) care was provided in a variety of ways. There were a mixture of both disease-specific services (dedicated stroke units) and generic disability services (mixed assessment/rehabilitation units) established within a variety of departments (general medicine, geriatric medicine,

---

Box 3.1   Categories of stroke care

- Dedicated stroke unit – disease-specific service such as a geographically defined ward or mobile team dedicated exclusively to the management of stroke patients.
- Mixed assessment/rehabilitation unit – generic disability service such as a ward or team focusing on the assessment and rehabilitation of disabling illness (including stroke).
- Acute admission unit – admits patients at the onset (within one week) of their illness.
- Delayed admission unit – admits patients after a delay of at least one week.
- General medical care – conventional care in general medical wards focusing on the management of acute medical illness but not on subsequent rehabilitation.

Adapted from Stroke Unit Trialists' Collaboration[6]

---

neurology, rehabilitation medicine). Ten of the units provided services which combined acute admission with a period of rehabilitation. In eight trials admission was delayed for at least one week and a period of ongoing rehabilitation was then provided. In one trial[22] admission occurred acutely but patients were discharged from the stroke unit after a few days.

The mixture of staff available was similar in both the organised (stroke unit) setting and the conventional care settings;[6] all included medical, nursing, and physiotherapy staff. Other staff commonly available for stroke care were occupational therapists (95% of stroke units vs 94% of conventional care), speech therapists (82% vs 88%), and social workers (82% vs 82%).

The main differences were apparent in the practice and organisation of care (Table 3.2). The organised (stroke unit) care was much more likely to include a co-ordinated multidisciplinary team, the routine involvement of carers, staffing by doctors/nurses with an interest in stroke and/or rehabilitation, the routine provision of information to patients and carers, and the provision of staff education programmes.

Co-ordinated multidisciplinary team care was defined as medical, nursing, and therapy staff being involved in stroke care and meeting formally at least on a weekly basis. Specialist staffing was considered to be present if the physicians and/or nurses had reported a special interest in stroke care and/or rehabilitation. Education and training included ongoing training programmes for staff in stroke. It is apparent from Table 3.2 that the procedures and

Table 3.1 Outline of stroke unit trials

Trial	Stroke patients	Comparison groups (organised vs conventional care)	Outcomes	Notes
Birmingham[8]	Within 2 weeks of stroke	Intensive rehabilitation in rehabilitation centre MARU (n=29) vs normal care in general wards (n=23)	Death and dependency at the end of follow-up (6–8 months)	Timing of outcomes not clear. Intervention not defined. 3 control patients lost to follow-up
Dover[9]	Within 9 weeks (most within 3 weeks) of stroke	DSU in stroke rehabilitation ward in geriatric medical unit (n=116) vs geriatric medicine MARU (n=28) or GMW (n=89)	Death, Rankin score, place of residence, length of hospital stay up to 1 year post-stroke	Minor randomisation imbalance. Numbers differ slightly from published report following re-analysis of original data
Edinburgh[10]	Acute patients (moderate severity) within 7 days of stroke	DSU in stroke rehabilitation ward in geriatric medicine (n=155) vs GMW (n=156)	Death, dependency, place of residence, length of hospital stay up to 1 year post-stroke	6 intervention and 10 control patients lost to follow-up
Goteburg-Ostra[11]	Acute patients within 7 days of stroke	Combined acute and rehabilitation DSU within general medical service (n=215) vs conventional care in GMW (n=202)	Death, Barthel score, place of residence, length of hospital stay	Not yet published
Goteborg-Sahlgren (unpublished)	Acute patients within 7 days of stroke	Combined acute and rehabilitation DSU neurology department vs conventional care in GMW	Death, Barthel score, place of residence, patient satisfaction, length of hospital stay up to 1 year	Not yet published
Helsinki[12]	Acute patients, over 65 years age, within 7 days of stroke	MARU in neurology ward (n=121) vs conventional care in GMW (n=122)	Death, Barthel and Rankin scores, length of hospital stay up to 1 year	Intention to treat data used (on treatment analysis gave more conservative result)
Illinois[13]	Within 1 year after stroke	MARU in rehabilitation centre (n=56) vs GMW (n=35) which had some specialist nursing input	Functional status and place of residence at end of follow-up	Poor definition of services. No death reported. RCT with 3:2 allocation to intervention:control

Table 3.1 continued

Trial	Stroke patients	Comparison groups (organised vs coventional care)	Outcomes	Notes
Kuopio[14]	Patients (at 7 days after stroke) able to tolerate intensive rehabilitation	DSU in neurological centre (n=50) vs GMW (n=45)	Death, ADL score, place of residence, duration of hosptal stay up to 1 year	Most patients screened failed to meet inclusion criteria for the trial
Montreal[15]	Acute patients within 7 days of stroke	DSU (mobile stroke team; n=65) vs conventional care in GMW (n=65)	Death, Barthel score, place of residence, length of initial hospital stay up to 6 weeks after stroke	Short follow-up period. 1 intervention and 3 control patients lost to follow-up
New York[16]	Within 2 months of stroke	MARU in rehabilitation centre (n=42) vs General wards (n=40) with some specialist nursing input	Functional status and place of residence at end of follow-up (approximately 1 year)	No deaths reported. Minor anomaly in published data table
Newcastle[17]	Acute patients (within 3 days of stroke)	MARU in geriatric medicine department (n=34) vs GMW (n=33)	Death, Barthel and Rankin scores, place of residence, length of hospital stay up to 6 months after stroke	Most patients screened did not meet trial inclusion criteria
Nottingham[18]	At 2 weeks after stroke	DSU (stroke rehabilitation ward) in geriatric medicine department (n=176) vs MARU in geriatric medicine department (n=63) or GMW (n=76)	Death, Barthel score, place of residence, length of hospital stay up to 6 months after stroke	Some crossover from GMW to geriatric medicine. RCT with 5:4 allocation to intervention:control
Orpington – 1993[19]	At 2 weeks after stroke	DSU (stroke rehabilitation ward) in geriatric medicine department (n=124) vs MARU in geriatric medicine department (n=73) or GMW (n=48)	Death, Barthel score, place of residence, length of hospital stay at end of follow-up	Variable duration of follow-up

Table 3.1 continued

Trial	Stroke patients	Comparison groups (organised vs coventional care)	Outcomes	Notes
Orpington – 1995[20]	Patients who have a poor prognosis at 2 weeks after stroke	DSU (stroke rehabilitiation ward) in geriatric medicine department (n = 36) vs GMW (n = 37)	Death, Barthel score, place of residence, length of hospital stay at end of follow-up	Variable duration of follow-up. 2 control patients lost to follow-up
Perth[21]	Within 7 days of stroke	Combined acute and rehabilitation DSU in neurology department (n = 28) vs GMW (n = 30)	Death, Barthel score, place of residence, length of hospital stay up to 6 months after stroke	Most patients screened did not enter trial
Tampere[22]	Within 7 days of stroke (usually earlier)	Acute, intensive DSU in neurology department (n = 98) vs MARU in a neurology department (n = 113)	Death, Rankin score, place of residence, length of hospital stay up to 1 year after stroke	Short duration (1 week) in DSU before transfer to conventional service
Trondheim[23]	Within 7 days (usually within 24 hours) of a stroke	Combined acute and rehabilitation DSU in general medical department (n = 110) vs GMW (n = 110)	Death, Barthel score, place of residence, length of stay in hospital or institution up to 1 year after stroke	Intention to treat data used
Umea[24]	Within 7 days of stroke	Combined acute rehabilitation DSU in general medical department (n = 110) vs GMW (n = 183)	Death, functional status, place of residence, length of initial hospital stay up to 1 year after stroke	Quasi-RCT (treatment allocation according to bed availability). One control patient lost to follow-up
Uppsala[25]	Patients admitted to general medical wards within 3 days of stroke	MARU (organised care within GMW; n = 60) vs conventional care in GMW (n = 52)	Death, ADL score, place of residence, length of stay in acute hospital up to 1 year after stroke	Quasi-RCT (treatment allocation according to admission rota)

Unless otherwise stated, all trials are RCTs with balanced allocation to intervention and control groups. Descriptions of service characteristics are provided in Box 3.1. Adapted from Stroke Unit Trialists' Collaboration.[6]
KEY: DSU, dedicated stroke unit (managing stroke patients only); MARU, mixed assessment/rehabilitation unit (managing other disabling illness as well as stroke); GMW, general medical ward; RCT, randomised controlled trial.

practices identified in the stroke unit trials very much reflected the concept of stroke unit care outlined in the past (Definitions of a stroke unit, Chapter 1, p 3).

Characteristics of different models of stroke unit

Having established the characteristic features of organised (stroke unit) care across all the trials (Table 3.2), we wished to establish that the different models of organised (stroke unit) care were sufficiently similar to justify combining them in the same analysis. In fact, the similarities were more striking than any differences. All the different models of stroke unit care incorporated specialist multidisciplinary team care co-ordinated through weekly meetings (Tables 3.3, 3.4) although some minor differences

Table 3.2 Characteristics of organised (stroke unit) care and conventional care

	Organised (stroke unit) care	Conventional care
Co-ordination of rehabilitation		
MDT care (weekly meetings)	All***	Some
Nursing practice integrated with MDT	All***	Some
Therapy practice integrated with MDT	All***	Some
Carers routinely involved in rehabilitation	Most***	Some
Carers routinely attend MDT meeting	Some*	Some
Specialisation of staff		
Physician interest in stroke	Most**	Some
Physician interest in rehabilitation	Most**	Some
Nursing interest in stroke	Most**	Some
Nursing interest in rehabilitation	Most***	Some
Education and training		
Routine information provision to carers	Most***	Some
Regular staff training	Most***	Some
Comprehensiveness of rehabilitation input		
Increased proportion of patients receive PT/OT	Most**	None
Earlier onset of PT/OT	Some**	None
Medical investigation/treatment protocols	Some*	None
Intensity of rehabilitation input		
More intensive PT/OT input	Some*	Some
Enhanced nurse:patient ratio	Some	Some

Results are expressed as the proportion of trials displaying specific characteristics (all descriptions are relative to the contemporary normal practice): all (100%), most (50–99%), some (1–49%), none (0%). The asterisk denotes the statistical significance of the difference between stroke unit and conventional care: *$p < 0.05$, **$p < 0.01$, ***$p < 0.001$. Key: PT, physiotherapy; OT, occupational therapy; MDT, multidisciplinary team. Derived from Table 2 of [6].

wcrc apparent:

- disease-specific units (dedicated stroke units) were more likely to be staffed by doctors and nurses who reported an interest in stroke whereas staff in generic disability services (mixed assessment/rehabilitation unit) were, not surprisingly, more likely to report an interest in rehabilitation (Table 3.3);
- acute admission units tended to be staffed by stroke specialists while delayed admission units employed rehabilitation specialists

Table 3.3   Characteristics of organised (stroke unit) care: dedicated stroke unit and mixed assessment/rehabilitation units

	Dedicated stroke unit (13 trials)	Mixed assessment/ rehabilitation unit (6 trials)
Admission and discharge policy		
Acute admission	Most	Most
Prolonged rehabilitation	Most	All
Disciplines routinely involved in stroke care		
Medical/nursing/PT	All	All
OT/SLT/social work	Most	Most
Co-ordination of rehabilitation		
MDT care (weekly meetings)	All***	All***
Nursing practice integrated with MDT	All***	All***
Therapy practice integrated with MDT	All***	All**
Carers routinely involved in rehabilitation	All***	Some
Carers routinely attend MDT meeting	Some*	Some
Specialisation of staff		
Physician interest in stroke	Most**	Some
Physician interest in rehabilitation	Most*	All*
Nursing interest in stroke	Most**	Some
Nursing interest in rehabilitation	Some	Most**
Education and training		
Routine information provision to carers	Most*	Some
Regular staff training	Most*	Some
Comprehensiveness of rehabilitation input		
Increased proportion of patients receive PT/OT	Most*	Some
Earlier onset of PT/OT	Some	Some
Medical investigation/treatment protocols	Some	Some
Intensity of rehabilitation input		
More intensive PT/OT input	Some	Some
Enhanced nurse:patient ratio	Some	Some

Results are expressed as the proportion of trials with a particular characteristic: all (100%), most (50–99%), some (1–49%), none (0%). The asterisk denotes whether the characteristic occurred more frequently than in the control (general medical wards) setting: *p < 0·05, **p < 0·01, ***p < 0·001. Key: PT, physiotherapy; OT, occupational therapy; SLT, speech & language therapy; MDT, multidisciplinary team.

(Table 3.4). Acute admission units were also more likely to use medical investigation and treatment protocols and to provide an earlier onset of physiotherapy and occupational therapy.

This descriptive information suggested that we had identified a group of trials comprising a variety of different models of organised (stroke unit) care which had in common certain basic character-istics: multidisciplinary organisation, staff specialisation, and education and training. However, it is important to recognise some methodological problems with our approach to analysing stroke unit services. Firstly, the information was obtained from the trialists who ran the stroke units; we were not able to obtain

Table 3.4 Characteristics of organised stroke unit care: acute or delayed admission

	Acute admission (11 trials)	Delayed admission (8 trials)
Admission and discharge policy		
Acute admission	All	None
Prolonged rehabilitation	Most	All
Disciplines routinely involved in stroke care		
Medical/nursing/PT	All	All
OT/SLT/social work	Most	Most
Co-ordination of rehabilitation		
MDT care (weekly meetings)	All***	All***
Nursing practice integrated with MDT	All***	All**
Therapy practice integrated with MDT	All***	All**
Carers routinely involved in rehabilitation	All***	Most
Carers routinely attend MDT meeting	Some	None
Specialisation of staff		
Physician interest in stroke	All***	Most**
Physician interest in rehabilitation	Most*	All**
Nursing interest in stroke	Most*	Most
Nursing interest in rehabilitation	Most**	All**
Education and training		
Routine information provision to carers	All***	Most**
Regular staff training	All***	Most*
Comprehensiveness of rehabilitation input		
Increased proportion of patients receive PT/OT	Some	Some
Earlier onset of PT/OT	Most**	Some
Medical investigation/treatment protocols	Most*	Some
Intensity of rehabilitation input		
More intensive PT/OT input	Some	Some
Enhanced nurse:patient ratio	Some	Some

Results and abbreviations are described with Table 3.3.

information from staff providing the conventional care. Therefore the findings may be biased by the expectation of the trialists as to which aspects of a stroke unit care may or may not be effective. Secondly, this was largely a retrospective analysis and in some cases the specific information was not available from the trialists or published reports. At best, the information in Tables 3.2–3.4 represents a strictly factual account of the service characteristics within the stroke unit trials. At the very worst, it represents a consensus view from the stroke unit trialists as to which features of stroke unit care were important. However, it does give us confidence that the trials we had identified were relatively consistent in certain core characteristics.

4: Effectiveness of organised (stroke unit) care

In this chapter, we describe the meta-analysis of those trials which compared organised inpatient (stroke unit) care with the contemporary conventional care. Patients receiving stroke unit care were more likely to survive, return home, and regain physical independence and there was an apparent reduction in secondary complications of stroke and an increase in the number of physically independent stroke survivors. Subgroup analyses did not indicate that any patient group, defined by gender, age or stroke severity, was likely to gain more or less benefit from stroke unit care. All stroke unit models which could provide a prolonged (weeks–months) period of multidisciplinary team care appeared to show benefit.

4.1 Conventions of meta-analysis

To address the most important question, "Are patients who receive organised inpatient (stroke unit) care more likely to have a good outcome than those receiving the contemporary conventional care?", we will use a technique termed "meta-analysis".

What is meta-analysis?

Meta-analysis is a statistical process for combining data from different trials. The simplest way to summarise the outcomes from a group of trials would entail adding together the results from the treatment group of each trial, adding together the control group results from each trial, and comparing these two grand totals.[1] In some circumstances this simple analysis may provide a useful description of the effects of a treatment. However, this approach cannot cope with trials where the treatment and control groups differ in size (i.e. the groups are not balanced by a 1:1

randomisation). A more flexible approach is to calculate odds ratios for the results of individual trials and for groups of trials.

What is an odds ratio?

An odds ratio is the ratio of the odds (the chance) of a particular outcome occurring amongst patients receiving the intervention in comparison with the corresponding odds (chance) of that outcome occurring amongst control patients. Odds ratios are normally expressed in terms of the prevention of a bad outcome. Therefore unity (odds ratio = 1) indicates an identical odds (chance) of a particular outcome occurring in the treatment and control groups and an odds ratio of < 1 indicates better outcomes in the intervention group. The calculated odds ratio is always an imperfect estimate of the "true" value and so is shown with its 95% confidence interval, which can be considered as the range of results with which this estimate of the odds ratio is reasonably compatible. Results can also be expressed as the odds reduction which reports the percentage reduction in the odds ratio resulting from treatment. Therefore, an odds ratio of 0.8 can be expressed as a 20% odds reduction.

If we consider an experiment where two coins ("intervention" coin A and "control" coin B) were each tossed 30 times, the odds (chance) of a "heads" appearing should be identical for each coin (i.e. odds ratio = 1). In fact, in this example coin A landed 14 "heads" and 16 "tails"; coin B landed 17 "heads" and 13 "tails". Therefore the odds ratio for landing "heads" with coin A (as opposed to coin B) is:

$$\text{Odds ratio} = 14/16 \text{ divided by } 17/13 = 0.67$$

This result appears very far from the expected value of 1 but a simple calculation[2] of the 95% confidence interval indicates that the "true" value could possibly lie in the range 0.24–1.85. The corresponding odds reduction is $100 \times (1 - 0.67) = 33\%$.

There are several different ways of calculating odds ratios and confidence intervals,[3,4] each having their advantages and disadvantages. The "fixed effect model"[3] is a standard approach in the UK but may be unreliable when the results of individual trials differ greatly from each other (i.e. there is heterogeneity). The alternative "random effects model"[4] can cope better with heterogeneity but tends to over-emphasise the influence of small trials. In practice, if odds ratios obtained with one statistical method are confirmed by other methods, this increases our confidence in the results.

| Comparison: | Tossing two coins | | | |
| Outcome: | Heads scores | | | |
Study	Expt n/N	Ctrl n/N	OR (95%CI Fixed)	OR (95%CI Fixed)
5 Tosses	4/5	2/5		6.00 [0.35, 101.57]
10 Tosses	6/10	3/10		3.50 [0.55, 22.30]
15 Tosses	7/15	8/15		0.77 [0.18, 3.21]
30 Tosses	14/30	17/30		0.67 [0.24, 1.85]
100 Tosses	53/100	45/100		1.38 [0.79, 2.40]
200 Tosses	106/200	97/200		1.20 [0.81, 1.77]
Total (95% CI)	**190/360**	**172/360**		**1.22 [0.91, 1.63]**

Figure 4.1   Coin tossing experiments. Six experiments were carried out in which an experimental and control coin was each tossed on a number of occasions. The figure shows the number (n) of occasions a "heads" was registered out of a total number (N) of tosses. The odds ratio from each experiment is expressed as a black box and the horizontal line represents the 95% confidence interval. The larger the black box, the greater the statistical power of the experiment. The diamond represents the odds ratio and 95% confidence interval of a meta-analysis of all six experiments. Further details in the text.

Presentation of results

By convention the results of each trial are presented as a black square with a horizontal line (Figure 4.1). The black square represents the odds ratio calculated for that individual trial and the horizontal line shows the 95% confidence interval. The summary result for a group of trials is shown as a diamond where the centre of the diamond indicates the summary odds ratio and the breadth of the diamond indicates the 95% confidence interval of that ratio.

We repeated the coin tossing example six times, each with a different number of coin tosses to represent six clinical trials (left hand column, Figure 4.1) with different numbers of patients. Coin A represented the intervention (experimental) group and coin B the controls. An adverse event was defined as landing "heads" and the total number of patients represented by the total number of coin tosses. The number of patients experiencing an adverse event (n) relative to the total number of patients (N) in the experimental group are shown in the second (Expt) column and similar data are provided for the controls in the third (Ctrl) column. The odds ratio and 95% confidence intervals for individual experiments and for groups of experiments are shown graphically while the right hand side of the figure displays the data numerically. It is conventional not only to list individual trials but to provide information on summary results (termed "subtotals") of groups of trials. At the bottom of each figure is the summary result ("Total") for all available trials.

In our (real) example we can see that none of the coin tossing experiments gave the expected odds ratio of 1 but the larger experiments tended to give more precise estimates (i.e. with narrower confidence intervals) and the summary result ("Total") was closest to the "true" answer.

(*Note:* We have presented a simplified meta-analysis figure. Often they will include other statistical data but the basic principle remains the same.)

Coping with different types of outcome

The meta-analysis method outlined above is designed to calculate the summary results for dichotomous outcomes, that is, outcomes which can be clearly split into two groups, for example alive or dead, persisting disability or no persisting disability. A number of other techniques are available to analyse continuous outcomes where the individual trials have reported the mean and standard deviation of a result such as a disability score or length of stay in hospital. In these approaches it is usual to calculate the difference between the mean result in the treatment and control groups and to calculate some summary (average) difference between treatment and control across all the various trials. Further information on these techniques is available elsewhere.[2]

Meta-analysis of the stroke unit trials

We can now use data from the stroke unit trials to carry out a meta-analysis in which we are asking the question, "Are patients who received organised inpatient (stroke unit) care less likely to have a bad outcome (more likely to have a good outcome) than those receiving the contemporary conventional care?". This question can be asked of different outcomes (for instance, death, disability) and within different groups of patients and different groups of trials.

Can the risk of death be reduced?

If stroke unit care is effective in reducing deaths then the majority of trials will show a reduction in deaths in the stroke unit group and the summary result will indicate a reduction in deaths overall. Figure 4.2 shows the results at the end of scheduled follow-up (a median of one year after stroke) in all the stroke unit trials for which results were available. The main comparison is organised stroke unit care versus the contemporary conventional care.

Three important points are apparent from Figure 4.2:

1. The confidence intervals of individual trials almost always include unity (odds ratio = 1), indicating that no result was statistically significant in its own right. However;
2. the great majority of trials observed fewer deaths among patients managed within the organised stroke unit care setting than in the conventional service. Therefore;

Comparison:	Organised stroke unit care vs conventional care			
Outcome:	Death by the end of scheduled follow-up			
Study	Expt n/N	Ctrl n/N	OR (95%CI Fixed)	OR (95%CI Fixed)
Birmingham	4/29	2/23		1.68 [0.28, 10.10]
Dover	39/116	46/117		0.78 [0.46, 1.33]
Edinburgh	48/155	55/156		0.82 [0.51, 1.32]
Goteborg (Ostra)	16/215	12/202		1.27 [0.59, 2.76]
Helsinki	26/121	27/122		0.96 [0.52, 1.77]
Illinois	0/56	0/35		0.63 [0.01, 32.39]
Kuopio	8/50	10/45		0.67 [0.24, 1.87]
Montreal	16/65	21/65		0.68 [0.32, 1.47]
New York	0/42	0/40		0.95 [0.02, 49.17]
Newcastle	11/34	12/33		0.84 [0.30, 2.30]
Nottingham	25/176	26/139		0.72 [0.39, 1.31]
Orpington (1993)	9/124	19/121		0.42 [0.18, 0.97]
Orpington (1995)	7/36	17/37		0.28 [0.10, 0.81]
Perth	4/29	6/30		0.64 [0.16, 2.55]
Tampere	30/98	27/113		1.41 [0.76, 2.58]
Trondheim	27/110	36/110		0.67 [0.37, 1.21]
Umea	43/110	75/183		0.92 [0.57, 1.50]
Uppsala	27/60	26/52		0.82 [0.39, 1.72]
Total (95%CI)	**340/1626**	**417/1623**		**0.81 [0.68, 0.96]**

Figure 4.2   Organised (stroke unit) care versus conventional care: death by the end of follow-up. Results of individual stroke unit trials are presented as the odds of death occurring by the end of scheduled follow-up (median 1 year: range 6 weeks – 1 year) in the stroke unit versus conventional care settings. The odds ratio and 95% confidence intervals of individual trials are presented as a black box and horizontal line. The pooled odds ratio and 95% confidence interval for all available trials is represented by the black diamond.

3. the summary (average) result across all the available trials indicated that patients receiving stroke unit care were less likely to die than those receiving the contemporary conventional care.

In fact, the summary result (odds ratio 0.81; 95% confidence interval 0.68–0.96) indicates that overall there was an 19% reduction in the chances of death but that the true result is likely to lie anywhere between a 4% and 32% reduction. The inconsistencies between different trials (i.e. the heterogeneity) were no more than would be expected by chance and several different ways of analysing the trials did not substantially alter the results.[5]

Why were deaths reduced?

The observation that patients managed in an organised stroke unit setting had a lower risk of death was surprising because interventions such as the organisation and delivery of rehabilitation were not expected to influence mortality after stroke. We were therefore interested to explore this observation further to try to establish why fewer deaths may have occurred in the stroke unit group. We first examined the pattern of deaths during the first year after the index stroke (i.e. the stroke event which resulted in the patient being recruited into a trial). Figure 4.3 shows the proportion (%) of patients who were known to have died within the stroke unit and control groups at various intervals after their index

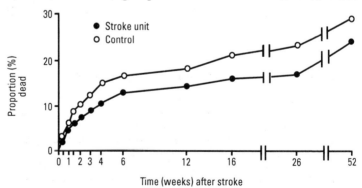

Figure 4.3 Organised (stroke unit) care versus conventional care (control): patterns of death after stroke. Results are presented as the proportion of patients for whom data were available who were known to be dead at specific census times after stroke. Adapted from the Stroke Unit Trialists' Collaboration[26].

stroke. A rapid rise in the number of deaths in both groups was apparent during the first six weeks but thereafter the death rate declined. The apparent difference in death rate between the stroke unit and control groups largely developed between one and three weeks after the index stroke and thereafter the risk of dying was very similar in the two groups. This is of particular interest because the period between one and three weeks is when most medical complications are believed to occur after stroke[6,7] and when most deaths are attributable to complications.[6] Many of these complications such as chest infections, urine infections, deep venous thrombosis, and pulmonary embolism, could conceivably be influenced by factors such as the identification of dysphagia, management of feeding, patient positioning, avoidance of urinary catheters, early mobilisation, and the prompt use of antibiotics or thromboprophylaxis. In contrast, deaths occurring very early (0–7 days) or late (weeks–months) after stroke tend to be due to direct neurological effects of the stroke and recurrent vascular events respectively.[6] These might not be expected to be influenced by stroke unit care.

We were able to further pursue the question of why deaths were reduced by examining the registered causes of deaths within the original trials. Unfortunately, data on the certified cause of death are often incomplete and not supported by more reliable information from postmortem examination. We did obtain death certificate information from 12 stroke unit trials (1611 patients) and grouped the deaths into four pre-specified categories of cause of death (Box 4.1).

Box 4.1   Classification of cause of death

Neurological – deaths attributable to the original (index) stroke or to a recurrent stroke. Examples include stroke, cerebral infarction, brain herniation, cerebral oedema or recurrent stroke.

Cardiovascular – examples include myocardial infarction, congestive cardiac failure, cardiac arrhythmia, and cardiac arrest.

Complications of immobility – any death which might reasonably be considered a complication of immobility. Examples would include infection (particularly of the chest or urinary tract), venous thromboembolism, decubitus ulceration.

Other causes – miscellaneous other illnesses, for example malignancy.

Adapted from the classification of Bamford *et al.*[6]

Table 4.1   Certified cause of death in the stroke unit trials

Category	Stroke unit	Control	Odds ratio (95% CI)
Neurological	9%	10%	0·9 (0·7–1·3)
Cardiovascular	5%	7%	0·7 (0·5–1·1)
Complications of immobility	4%	6%	0·6 (0·4–1·0)
Other causes	4%	4%	0·9 (0·5–1·5)

Results are presented as the proportion (%) of patients in the stroke unit and control groups who died with a particular category of (certified) cause of death. The odds ratio (95% confidence interval) shows the chance (odds) of a stroke unit patient dying of a particular cause in comparison with a patient in the conventional care (control) setting. Adapted from Stroke Unit Trialists' Collaboration.[26]

The proportion of stroke unit and control group patients within particular categories of cause of death are shown in Table 4.1. Although we have been able to combine information from several trials, this analysis still lacks sufficient information (statistical power) to draw really convincing conclusions. A fair conclusion might be that the trend towards fewer deaths in the stroke unit group was apparent across all four cause of death categories but was most marked for those considered to be due to either complications of immobility or cardiovascular disease.

Preventing death at the expense of increased dependency amongst survivors?

Our results indicate that organised (stroke unit) care may reduce the risk of death after stroke although these findings are not beyond reasonable doubt. However, if deaths really have been reduced, can we be confident that this has been of overall benefit to the patients? Concerns have been expressed[8] that some new treatments for stroke patients might prevent deaths but at the expense of causing more morbidity, such that patients will be kept alive only to suffer prolonged periods of severe disability. To be confident that stroke unit care is of overall benefit, we need to establish whether patients are more likely to experience a "good" outcome (regain independence, return home) if they are managed in a stroke unit setting. There are two relatively simple ways in which we can examine this question.

We could look at the number of patients who either died or required long term institutional care (in a hospital, nursing home or residential home). These outcomes are easy to define and are robust in that there is likely to be no doubt as to whether a patient is alive and living in their own home or in a nursing home.

However, reduced institutionalisation could simply reflect improved discharge planning rather than reduced dependency (disability). Also, there may be no consistent relationship across the trials between the level of dependency and the risk of institutionalisation.

We could analyse the number of patients who either died or were known to be physically dependent. This is a more direct measure of what we want to know but is potentially subject to detection bias; if the research worker who assesses the patients' level of dependency is aware of whether the patient was managed in the stroke unit or control setting, this may influence the way in which they judge the level of dependency (see Systematic error (bias), Chapter 2, p 12).

Clearly, both approaches to measuring morbidity within the stroke unit trials have their advantages so we shall describe both sets of results.

Is the need for institutional care reduced?

Figure 4.4 summarises the stroke unit trial results in terms of the combined poor outcome of a patient being either dead or requiring long term institutional care. These were measured at the end of scheduled follow-up (median of one year after stroke). If we first look at the odds ratios and confidence intervals for individual trials we can see that a number of studies[9-13] observed impressive reductions in poor outcomes among the stroke unit patients. In a further 11 trials there were less convincing reductions. The summary result for all trials is consistent with a highly significant (odds ratio 0.75; 95% CI 0.65–0.87; 2p<0.0001) reduction in poor outcomes. In this case, however, the results of individual trials varied from each other rather more than might be expected by chance and so an alternative statistical model (random effects model) was used to assess the results. This produced a very similar result (odds ratio 0.74; 95% CI 0.62–0.89; 2p<0.0001). Some of the variation between the individual trials may have been due to the different periods of follow-up because trials with a short follow-up period are likely to find more patients still resident in hospital or rehabilitation clinics. Re-analysis of the results including only trials with a prolonged period of follow-up (six months or one year) produced very similar results (odds ratio 0.76; 95% CI 0.64–0.90; 2p<0.01) with much less heterogeneity apparent between trials.

The observed reduction in the combined poor outcome of death or requirement for institutional care is statistically very robust. We can calculate that we would have to identify unpublished neutral trials (odds ratio = 1) containing over 4000 randomised patients to overturn this result. Our findings indicate that the improved survival among stroke unit patients was not at the expense of more patients requiring institutional care and that the reduced need for institutional care was not due to unreasonable hospital discharge policies because the benefits were sustained for a period of up to one year after stroke (Figure 4.4).

Is dependency (disability) among survivors reduced?

While the requirement for long term care is a reasonably useful surrogate for disability[14] which is unlikely to be subject to detection bias, the absolute rates of institutionalisation will be influenced by national and cultural factors. Although a reduced need for

Comparison:	Organised stroke unit care vs conventional care			
Outcome:	Death or institutional care by the end of scheduled follow-up			
Study	Expt n/N	Ctrl n/N	OR (95%CI Fixed)	OR (95%CI Fixed)
Dover	61/116	66/117		0.86 [0.51, 1.44]
Edinburgh	66/155	78/156		0.74 [0.47, 1.16]
Goteborg (Ostra)	49/215	43/202		1.09 [0.69, 1.74]
Helsinki	36/121	46/122		0.70 [0.41, 1.19]
Illinois	22/56	17/35		0.69 [0.29, 1.61]
Kuopio	22/50	23/45		0.74 [0.33, 1.69]
Montreal	57/65	52/65		1.78 [0.68, 4.64]
New York	15/42	17/40		0.75 [0.31, 1.83]
Newcastle	18/34	21/33		0.64 [0.24, 1.71]
Nottingham	62/176	53/139		0.88 [0.56, 1.40]
Orpington (1993)	33/124	52/121		0.48 [0.28, 0.82]
Orpington (1995)	18/36	30/37		0.23 [0.08, 0.67]
Perth	6/29	14/30		0.30 [0.09, 0.94]
Tampere	43/98	42/113		1.32 [0.76, 2.30]
Trondheim	41/110	61/110		0.48 [0.28, 0.82]
Umea	51/110	105/183		0.64 [0.40, 1.03]
Uppsala	40/60	35/52		0.97 [0.44, 2.14]
Total (95% CI)	**640/1597**	**755/1600**		**0.75 [0.65, 0.87]**

Figure 4.4 Organised (stroke unit) care versus conventional care: death or institutionalisation at the end of scheduled follow-up. Results are presented as the odds ratio (95% confidence interval) of the combined adverse outcome of being dead or requiring institutional care at the end of scheduled follow-up (median 1 year: range 6 weeks – 1 year). Abbreviations and terms are as Figure 4.2.

institutional care could be of some economic interest, it is of less profound significance than the possibility that fewer patients were remaining dependent. Therefore, our third outcome measure was to look at the total number of patients who were known to be dead or physically dependent at the end of scheduled follow-up. However, this analysis raised two major problems.

Physical dependency was measured in different ways within different trials and so we had to establish comparable measures of dependency across the different trials. In fact, almost all the primary trials had used some form of dependency score and we could define a patient as being dependent if they required help with walking, transfers, dressing, washing or eating. Using these criteria and with the help of the original trialists, it was possible to establish how many survivors were "independent" or "dependent". The chosen value to indicate physical independence was equivalent to a Rankin score of 0–2 or a Barthel index of more than 18/20 (Box 4.2). Dependent patients had equivalent to a Rankin score[15] of 3–5 or Barthel index[15] of 0–18/20.

There was a risk of detection bias. Therefore, we analysed the results for all available trials and then for a subgroup of trials which had clearly used a "blinded" research worker to assess outcome.

Figure 4.5 outlines the results for all those trials comparing organised (stroke unit) care with the contemporary conventional care analysed as the combined poor outcome of being dead or physically dependent at the end of scheduled follow-up (median one year). In all but one trial the stroke unit group were less likely to be dead or physically dependent at the end of follow-up than those managed in a conventional care setting. The summary result for all the available trials indicated that there was a highly significant reduction in this poor outcome, with an odds ratio of

---

Box 4.2   Independence defined on Barthel and Rankin measures

Barthel index 19–20	Able to wash, toilet, transfer, dress, walk independently Continent of urine and faeces May need help with stairs or bathing
Rankin Scale 0–2	None or slight disability Able to look after own affairs without assistance

0.71 (95% CI 0.61–0.84; 2p<0.0001). The results of the individual trials varied slightly more than might be expected by chance but once again a re-analysis using an alternative (random effects) statistical model produced very similar results (OR 0.72; 95% CI 0.61–0.83; 2p<0.0001). The results were not altered by excluding trials with different periods of follow-up, different randomisation procedures or looking at different models of stroke unit care.

We have indicated the concerns about the degree of "blinding" of the outcome assessment. The odds ratio for death or dependency within the five trials[13,16–19] which used an unequivocally blinded outcome assessment on all patients (OR 0.72; 95% CI 0.55–0.94; 2p<0.01) was almost identical to the results for all available trials. This gives us some confidence that the results of the systematic review are not solely due to a detection bias.

Comparison:	Organised stroke unit care vs conventional care			
Outcome:	Death or dependency by the end of scheduled follow-up			
Study	Expt n/N	Ctrl n/N	OR (95%CI Fixed)	OR (95%CI Fixed)
Birmingham	8/29	9/23		0.59 [0.18, 1.91]
Dover	65/116	79/117		0.61 [0.36, 1.04]
Edinburgh	93/155	94/156		0.99 [0.63, 1.56]
Helsinki	47/121	65/122		0.56 [0.33, 0.93]
Illinois	20/56	17/35		0.59 [0.25, 1.39]
Kuopio	31/50	31/45		0.74 [0.31, 1.73]
Montreal	58/65	60/65		0.69 [0.21, 2.30]
New York	23/42	23/40		0.89 [0.37, 2.14]
Newcastle	26/34	28/33		0.58 [0.17, 2.00]
Nottingham	123/176	100/139		0.91 [0.55, 1.48]
Orpington (1993)	101/124	108/121		0.53 [0.25, 1.10]
Orpington (1995)	34/34	37/37		0.92 [0.02, 47.65]
Perth	10/29	14/30		0.60 [0.21, 1.72]
Tampere	53/98	55/113		1.24 [0.72, 2.14]
Trondheim	54/110	81/110		0.35 [0.20, 0.61]
Umea	52/110	102/183		0.71 [0.44, 1.14]
Uppsala	45/60	41/52		0.80 [0.33, 1.95]
Total (95%CI)	843/1409	944/1421		0.71 [0.60, 0.84]

Figure 4.5 Organised (stroke unit) care versus conventional care: death or dependency at the end of scheduled follow-up. Results are presented as the odds ratio (95% confidence interval) of the combined adverse outcome of death or dependency at the end of scheduled follow-up (median 1 year: range 6 weeks – 1 year). Abbreviations and terms are as Figure 4.2.

Is quality of life among survivors improved?

We would hope that an effective intervention which could improve a patient's objective outcomes such as survival or disability would also enhance their subjective health status or quality of life. Unfortunately, this outcome is difficult to define and measure and was recorded in only two trials (Indredavik B *et al*, 8th Nordic Meeting on Cerebrovascular Diseases, August 1995, Trondheim, Norway;[19]). Both trials found a pattern of improved quality of life in the stroke unit survivors.

What are the absolute benefits of stroke unit care?

So far we have examined the results of the stroke unit trials in terms of the three primary outcomes: death, death or requiring institutional care and death or physical dependency. The approach we have outlined is that of relative outcome rates where the results among patients randomised to the intervention group are expressed relative to the results in patients randomised to the control group (for example, using an odds ratio). This approach is statistically robust but can be difficult to interpret. It is therefore of interest to look also at the absolute outcome rates where we can express results simply as the proportion (%) of patients in each outcome group at the end of scheduled follow-up or use more sophisticated measures such as the risk difference which take into account variations between individual trials (Table 4.2). We can express the absolute benefits in one of at least two ways.

Results can be calculated in terms of the number of adverse

Table 4.2   Absolute outcomes in the stroke unit trials

Outcome	Stroke unit	Control	Odds ratio (95% CI)	Absolute difference in outcomes (95% CI)
Home (independent)	39%	33%	1.4 (1.2–1.7)	+5 (+1–+8)
Home (dependent)	18%	16%	1·0 (0·7–1·4)	0 (−4–+3)
Institutional care	20%	22%	0·8 (0·7–1·0)	−1 (−4–+1)
Dead	23%	28%	0·8 (0·7–1·0)	−4 (−7–0)

The table shows the proportion (%) of patients in the stroke unit and control groups who were in each outcome category at the end of scheduled follow-up (median one year). Also shown is the odds rato (95% CI) of a particular outcome occurring in the stroke unit versus control group and the absolute difference (95% CI) in outcomes per 100 patients treated calculated from the risk difference. The terms "independent" and "dependent" are described in Box 4.2. Adapted from Stroke Unit Trialists' Collaboration.[26]

outcomes avoided by managing 100 patients in an organised (stroke unit) care setting. It is apparent in Table 4.2 that for every 100 patients managed in a stroke unit, five more returned home in an independent state, four fewer died, and one less was in institutional care. Therefore stroke unit care was associated with an absolute increase in "good" outcomes without any substantial increase in the number of dependent survivors, living either at home or in an institution.

Results can be calculated as the numbers who need to be managed in an organised stroke unit to prevent one adverse outcome;[20] the number needed to treat (NNT). Using data in Table 4.2, we can calculate that approximately 25 (95% CI 14–infinity) patients need to be treated to prevent one death, while the NNT to ensure one extra patient returns home independent is 20 (95%CI 13–100). These results compare favourably with many medical interventions.[20] This information can be used to carry out an economic analysis of stroke unit care (Chapter 5).

The results presented in this chapter strongly suggest that stroke unit care can be effective. However, in Chapter 3 (Defining the patient group, p 21) we outlined a number of other controversial issues, one of which was which patients can benefit from organised stroke unit care? It had previously been suggested[21] that stroke unit care was most suitable for a "middle band" of stroke patients who had residual disability but were not so unwell as to be unable to co-operate with rehabilitation. It had also been common practice to exclude certain groups of patients such as the elderly from stroke units in the belief that they would benefit less. At the onset of this systematic review we identified certain patient subgroups we wished to examine, looking for evidence that certain groups would gain more or less benefit than others. However, before doing so we must first acknowledge the limitations and potential hazards of carrying out this kind of "subgroup analysis" (Box 4.3).

Subgroup analysis

Subgroup analysis involves the recalculation of the results of a trial or meta-analysis focusing on one section (subgroup) of the study. Subgroup analysis can provide useful information to guide clinical practice and to explain differences between different trials. For example, the benefit gained from aspirin or cholesterol lowering therapy is more apparent in individuals at high risk of vascular disease than in those at low risk.[1,22] However, subgroup

---

Box 4.3   Questions to ask about subgroup analyses[25]

1. Subgroup analyses of a small number of hypotheses stated in advance?
2. Difference between subgroups consistent across studies?
3. Difference between subgroups clinically and statistically significant?
4. Other supporting indirect evidence?

---

analysis can frequently produce inaccurate, misleading results[23,24] and the greater the number of analyses, the greater the risk of generating a spurious result. Therefore, all subgroup analyses should be treated with caution and before accepting the results, we should consider the following questions.[25]

Was the analysis based on one of a small number of hypotheses stated in advance? Subgroup analyses carried out after the event to explain untidy results are particularly susceptible to bias and spurious results.[25] At best, they should be used to generate hypotheses for future research. We therefore restricted our analysis to a few pre-specified subgroup questions.

Was the difference between subgroups consistent across studies? Subgroup analyses which have compared the results in one group of patients tested in one trial with another group of patients in a different trial will be comparing not only patient groups but also all the other differences between the two trials. However, if the subgroup data are available across a range of studies one can be more confident that they provide a valid comparison of the subgroups of interest. We were able to obtain subgroup data for the majority of trials including at least 2000 patients.

Was the difference between subgroups clinically and statistically significant? Any apparent subgroup differences should be interpreted cautiously in the light of their statistical and clinical meaning. Although data were available from 2000 patients this represents a relatively small amount of information.

Is there other indirect evidence to support the apparent difference between subgroups? Corroborative evidence from, for example, animal studies may support the subgroup hypothesis although there is a danger that biologically plausible (but incorrect) theories are easy to develop. Unfortunately, much of rehabilitation practice cannot usefully draw upon corroborative evidence from the basic sciences.

Which patients benefit?

Bearing in mind these limitations, we examined the results from the stroke unit trials divided into three subgroups defined by patient characteristics:

1. *Gender* – male, female
2. *Age* – <75 years, ⩾75 years
3. *Stroke severity* – at the outset of the systematic review we categorised initial stroke severity within the stroke unit trials according to three broad criteria:
   - mild stroke – patient able to stand (with or without assistance) at the time of randomisation (this is approximately equivalent to achieving a Barthel index of at least 10/20 during the first week after stroke);
   - moderate stroke – functional abilities intermediate between mild and severe;
   - severe stroke – patient does not have sitting balance at the time of randomisation (approximately equivalent to a Barthel index of <3/20 during the first week after stroke).

Figure 4.6 outlines the results for the patient subgroups in terms of

Comparison:	Organised stroke unit care vs conventional care		
Outcome:	Death or institutional care by the end of follow-up		
Subgroup	Expt n/N	Ctrl n/N	OR (95% CI Fixed)
Sex			
Female	172/418	193/384	
Male	120/366	158/364	
Age			
<75 years	241/839	273/796	
⩾75 years	202/398	290/472	
Initial stroke severity			
mild	36/287	47/273	
Moderate	279/649	317/627	
Severe	179/229	199/232	

Figure 4.6 Organised (stroke unit) care versus conventional care: analysis of patient subgroups. Results are presented as the odds ratio (95% confidence interval) of the combined adverse outcome of death or requiring long term institutional care. Definitions of stroke severity are given in the text. (Adapted from Stroke Unit Trialists' Collaboration[5])

the combined poor outcome of being dead or requiring long term institutional care. There are relatively few data available in each subgroup, which limits the statistical power of these analyses. However, within the limitations of these data the effectiveness of stroke unit care did not appear to vary with the patients' age, gender or stroke severity. It is important to recognise that the majority of stroke unit trials incorporated some selection criteria according to stroke severity and so had already excluded some patients with very mild and very severe strokes from the group which we stratified into mild, moderate, and severe categories. We therefore cannot comment on the effectiveness of stroke unit care for the mildest or severest stroke patients.

The results presented in Figure 4.6 show the relative reduction in poor outcomes in a stroke unit group as opposed to those managed in conventional care. We can also look at the absolute outcome rates in terms of the proportion (%) of patients within each outcome group. These results[26] indicate that the patients with the mild strokes gained no benefit in terms of increased survival but more of the survivors regained physical independence. Approximately 25 mild stroke patients need to be treated to produce one extra physically independent survivor (NNT 25). The moderate stroke group appeared to benefit in terms of an increase in the proportion who survived (NNT 33) and an increase in the proportion who survived in a physically independent state (NNT 17). The patients with the severest strokes showed the greatest apparent benefit from stroke unit care in terms of survival (NNT 17) and a small (but statistically non-significant) increase in the proportion of independent survivors (NNT 100). All the estimates are imprecise with confidence intervals which include the possibility of no benefit.

The main conclusion which can be drawn from these subgroup analyses is that all categories of patients recruited into the stroke unit trials appeared to benefit from stroke unit care and there are no firm grounds to exclude patients on the basis of gender, age or (within the limits of patients recruited into the trials) stroke severity.

What kind of stroke unit is effective?

In this systematic review we have identified randomised trials comparing two broad and ill defined systems of care: a stroke unit "black box" and a conventional care "black box". This initial comparison has allowed us to conclude that improvements in the organisation of inpatient stroke care can bring about important improvements in the recovery of patients and that the nihilism which has previously surrounded stroke care is unjustified. However, although these are important conclusions they only represent a first step towards delivering better stroke care. These simple conclusions conceal the underlying diversity and complexity of the individual trials and the systems of care which they were comparing. As this review is essentially a pragmatic exercise to identify reliable information to guide the care of individual stroke patients, we must explore the diversity within the individual trials. However, there is a paradox: by asking increasingly more specific questions by carrying out "subgroup analyses", we are likely to produce more statistically unreliable answers (Box 4.3).

Exploring the diversity of stroke unit trials

Broadly speaking, there are two approaches we can use to try to further explore the stroke unit trials and unpack the "black box" of stroke unit care. Firstly, we can extend the systematic review to look at the results obtained within subgroups of trials examining stroke units which had particular practices and procedures. In essence, this approach will identify the "average" stroke unit characteristics and is probably more useful for assessing broad questions of policy and procedure rather than for looking at specific details of stroke unit practice. The second approach, which might be considered a form of "mentorship", is to choose good examples of organised (stroke unit) care which have been tested within a randomised controlled trial. Using this approach, we could collect a series of case studies of stroke care providing specific examples of stroke unit practices and procedures. However, with this approach we abandon the systematic review and there is a danger that the information we get will be biased or idiosyncratic.

In our attempt to analyse the characteristics of stroke unit care, we have employed both the approaches outlined above: subgroup analyses to examine differences in policy and qualitative approaches to examine practices and procedures within chosen units (see Appendix). With the latter approach we have tried to obtain information from more than one source[27] using both published information and a structured interview with the trialists (Appendix). In describing the specific examples of stroke unit care, we have used both a detailed questionnaire and obtained descriptions of "vignettes" of care provided for hypothetical patients.

What general policies should be applied?

There are four broad questions concerning the organisation of inpatient stroke care which are of considerable practical importance and can be addressed through the stroke unit trials. These concern whether stroke units should:

1. comprise a geographically discrete ward or alternatively a mobile stroke team;
2. be established within a particular departmental setting;
3. organise the timing of admission and discharge in a particular way (i.e. early or delayed admission, early discharge or prolonged rehabilitation);
4. select only stroke patients or cater for a mixed disability group.

Stroke ward or mobile team

Do the apparent benefits of organised inpatient (stroke unit) care require a geographically defined stroke ward or can they be delivered by a mobile team providing care to patients in a variety of wards? Unfortunately, only one trial[18] has evaluated a mobile team. The procedures and practices of this team appeared to be very similar to those described in stroke wards but there are insufficient data to comment reliably on the effectiveness of such a team. We can be most confident about the effectiveness of geographically defined stroke wards.

Department setting

The systems of organised stroke care which have been studied in randomised trials were established in a variety of medical departments, including departments of geriatric medicine, general medicine, neurology, and rehabilitation medicine. Once again, it was apparent that there are considerable similarities between the different departmental settings. In particular, they all provided co-ordinated multidisciplinary team care with an increased likelihood of routinely involving carers in the rehabilitation process (unpublished observations) although conclusions are limited by the small number of trials in each subgroup. The differences that existed indicated a trend towards a more disease-specific approach within the departments of general medicine and neurology and a more generic disability approach within departments of geriatric medicine and rehabilitation medicine (unpublished observations). However, there was no evidence that better results were obtained with stroke units established within a particular departmental setting (Figure 4.7).

51

Admission and discharge policies

The admission and discharge policies of the stroke units are important considerations in the planning and delivery of a service. The stroke unit studies have employed a variety of admission and discharge policies with admission occurring either immediately after the stroke or after a delay of 1–2 weeks. Discharge policies have ranged from routine discharge within a week of the stroke[28] through to an unlimited duration of stay.[9–11,16–19,29–33] Intermediate policies included setting maximum limits of four,[34] six,[12] twelve,[13] or 16 weeks.[35] Within the stroke unit trials, 11 looked at systems incorporating an acute admission policy while eight incorporated a delayed admission policy.[5] As all but one of the trials were similar in offering some period of prolonged care, we have analysed the trials by their admission policy. We have previously (Table 3.4) outlined the main characteristics of those stroke units with an acute admission policy versus those with a policy of delaying admission for 1–2 weeks. These two types of service had very similar staffing characteristics and were much more likely to provide co-ordinated

Comparison: Organised stroke unit care vs conventional care Outcome: Death or institution care by the end of follow-up			
Subgroup	Expt n/N	Ctrl n/N	OR (95%CI Fixed)
Patient mix			
Mixed disability group	131/313	136/282	
Stroke patients only	397/1019	494/1041	
Admission policy			
Acute (≤7 days)	350/932	445/1001	
Delayed (>7 days)	233/600	258/534	
Maximum duration of intervention			
1 week	43/98	42/113	
4–16 weeks	311/744	396/798	
Unlimited	327/815	360/741	
Departmental setting			
General medicine	181/495	244/547	
Geriatric medicine	258/641	297/603	
Neurology	107/298	126/310	
Rehabilitation med.	37/98	34/75	

Figure 4.7 Organised (stroke unit) care versus conventional care: subgroup analysis by stroke unit characteristics. Results are presented as the odds ratio (95% confidence interval) of the combined adverse outcome of death or requiring long term institutional care. Definitions of stroke unit characteristics are given in the text. (Adapted from Stroke Unit Trialists' Collaboration[5])

multidisciplinary care than that which is conventionally available in general wards (Table 3.4). The differences between the two types of unit were minor and focused on the organisation of early medical and paramedical care (Table 3.4).

The results for both these sets of trials are shown in Figure 4.7. We can see that within the limitations of the data, both admission policies were associated with improved patient outcomes compared with those in general wards. Figure 4.7 also shows results for the discharge policies; one trial incorporated a short (one week) duration of care, six trials incorporated intermediate durations of care (maximum of between four and 16 weeks), and 12 trials did not set a limit on the duration of admission. It is clear from Figure 4.7 that all the current evidence regarding the effectiveness of organised (stroke unit) care has arisen from trials which have provided a duration of admission of at least several weeks.

Patient mix

Should stroke patients be admitted to disease-specific units only providing care for stroke patients (dedicated stroke unit) or can equally effective care be provided within generic disability services (mixed assessment/rehabilitation unit)? This is a question of considerable practical importance and relevance across a number of countries. Stroke care is commonly provided within mixed units; for example, geriatric medical assessment/rehabilitation wards particularly within the UK,[36] and neurology assessment/rehabilitation wards particularly in Scandinavia.[16]

We were able to use the stroke unit trials to explore these questions. Before doing so, it is important to recognise that these types of comparison can be either "indirect" (i.e. we can compare the results of trials of a dedicated unit vs general ward with trials of a mixed unit vs general ward). These are relatively unreliable because the different trials may vary in a whole range of ways. The more reliable comparison is a "direct" one (i.e. based on trials which have randomised patients to either dedicated stroke units or mixed units). Within this systematic review 11 trials (2060 patients) incorporated a comparison of a disease-specific dedicated stroke unit (with multidisciplinary care) with a general medical ward[37] and six trials (647 patients) directly compared a mixed assessment/rehabilitation unit (with multidisciplinary care) with a general medical ward.[5] In four trials (542 patients), patients were randomised to a direct comparison of a dedicated stroke unit with a mixed assessment/rehabilitation unit.[5]

The charactcristics of the dedicated stroke units and mixed rehabilitation units were similar (Table 3.3) in that they were likely to be staffed by individuals with a specialist interest in stroke care, provided co-ordinated multidisciplinary care, and offered a pro-longed period of input (with either immediate or delayed admission). The differences between the two models of care were relatively minor (Table 3.3).

Figure 4.8 shows the comparisons for the different types of care for the main outcome of death or requirement for institutional care. Both dedicated stroke units and mixed assessment/rehabilitation units tended to achieve better results, of similar magnitude, than general medical wards. Direct comparisons of a dedicated stroke unit versus a mixed assessment/rehabilitation unit (Figure 4.8) were hampered by the small patient numbers but did not indicate any significant difference between the two systems of organised care. Similar results were obtained when analysed on the combined outcome of being dead or physically dependent. We can therefore conclude that at present we have evidence to indicate that both disease-specific (dedicated stroke) units and generic disability (mixed assessment/rehabilitation) units which have developed co-ordinated multidisciplinary care can improve outcomes compared with those of general medical wards. When the two systems of organised care have been directly compared there is a trend towards better results in the dedicated stroke unit setting but these

Comparison:	Dedicated stroke unit vs mixed assessment/ rehabilitation unit		
Outcome:	Death or institutional care by the end of a scheduled follow-up		
Study	Expt n/N	Ctrl n/N	OR (95%CI Fixed)
Dover	11/18	18/28	
Nottingham (elderly)	34/78	32/63	
Orpington (1993)	24/71	33/73	
Tampere	43/98	42/113	
Total (95%CI)	112/265	125/277	

Figure 4.8 Direct comparison of dedicated stroke unit versus mixed assessment/rehabilitation unit. Results are presented as the odds ratio (95% confidence interval) of the combined adverse outcome of death or requiring institutional care by the end of scheduled follow-up.

results are not conclusive.

In our exploration of the best general policies we can therefore conclude the following.

- Both disease-specific dedicated stroke units and generic disability mixed assessment/rehabilitation units have been able to produce better results than conventional care in general medical wards.
- We cannot say at present whether one of these models is more effective than another.
- Units incorporating both immediate admission and admission delayed for 1–2 weeks have produced better results than general medical wards.
- All the available evidence of benefit comes from units which have been able to provide care for at least several weeks if necessary.
- Apparently successful stroke units have been established in a variety of departmental settings.
- All units shared certain procedures and practices in common.

Box 4.4   Summary of results

- Patients managed in a stroke unit were more likely to survive, regain independence, and return home.
- Benefits were not restricted to any subgroup of patients.
- Benefits were observed in several models of stroke unit care.

5: Economics of stroke unit care

In this economic analysis of the systematic review we examine whether stroke units are cost effective. The main costs of acute stroke are attributable to hospital care, whereas long term costs largely relate to the level of residual disability. Stroke unit care appears not only to improve patient outcomes but also reduce economic costs by freeing up resources for alternative uses. Within the limitations of this analysis stroke units are likely to be more cost effective than conventional care in general wards.

Economic analysis

Economic evaluations of health care interventions seek to identify, measure, and value the costs and benefits of two or more alternative courses of action. They are increasingly important because of the escalating cost of health care worldwide and the recognition that resources available are limited. Therefore we need to identify health care interventions which are not only effective but can also deliver the greatest benefit for the least cost.

Methods of economic analysis

We have summarised the evidence on the effectiveness of organised inpatient (stroke unit) care with respect to conventional care in general medical wards (Chapter 4). This chapter sets out an economic evaluation in which we:

- discuss the main determinants of the cost of stroke care;
- list the potential economic costs and benefits of introducing organised stroke unit care;
- examine the potential influence of stroke unit care on these costs and benefits;
- quantify these influences using independent external sources of economic data;
- explore the reliability of the underlying assumptions;
- provide an interpretation of the findings.

Terminology

Before we describe this evaluation, we need to explain a number of the commonly used terms.[1]

- The *effectiveness* of an intervention is the degree to which the desired outcomes are achieved in everyday practice. This differs from *efficacy* which is the impact in the ideal circumstances.
- The *efficiency* of an intervention expresses the number of beneficial outcomes (such as lives saved) divided by its cost in terms of money or resources. Therefore, economic efficiency is achieved when the maximum number of beneficial outcomes are obtained from a given budget.
- A *cost-effectiveness* analysis compares the cost of different ways of tackling the same health problem (for example, stroke unit versus general medical ward) by calculating the net number of beneficial outcomes different interventions will achieve divided by their cost.
- A *cost–benefit* analysis assesses the return on investment in terms of money. For example, what returns would be achieved by spending £100,000 on stroke care or renal dialysis?
- Costs are divided into two categories: *direct costs* include the direct use of services (such as drugs, nursing care), while *indirect costs* indicate losses such as loss of income or productivity.

Sources of data for economic analysis

None of the clinical trials discussed in the preceding chapters conducted an economic evaluation in parallel with the clinical research study (i.e. a primary economic evaluation). Consequently we must conduct a secondary evaluation using other data sources. While this is not as reliable as a primary evaluation, this approach has the advantage that we can use readily accessible data about stroke unit effectiveness which can be precise because it is based on large numbers of clinical trials. The disadvantages are that it assumes that the cost data will apply equally to a variety of settings.

Costs of stroke

In Chapter 1 we referred to the global burden of stroke disease. More detailed costings confirm this major economic burden of stroke. For example, within the United Kingdom, the direct cost per case to the National Health Service is very high. Isard and Forbes[2] used a "top-down" approach (i.e. dividing the total cost of stroke care by the number of cases of stroke) to calculate costs as being equivalent to £5827 per stroke case when updated to 1996–7 prices (Hospital and Community Services Pay and Prices Index, personal communication). To this we must add the cost of premature death and morbidity, loss of earnings and production, the use of social care, unpaid carer time, and other hidden costs. A more recent "bottom-up" analysis, where the individual components of the stroke cost are identified and aggregated (Forbes and Dennis, Scottish Office Report, 1995), produced an even higher estimate of £8536 per stroke case.

When discussing the costs of stroke care, we can divide them into those due to either acute or longer term care.

Acute stroke costs are largely attributable to hospital care[3] with the direct hospital costs (at least in the UK but probably also in other countries) being dominated by the costs of nursing care and hospital overheads[3] (Table 5.1). However, in other health care systems with a more technological approach toward stroke care, the balance of costs may be altered to some extent but the same principles are likely to apply. Therefore the main determinants of the direct costs of acute stroke care will relate closely to length of hospital stay.

Costs in the longer term are largely attributable to the care of dependent individuals in hospital or nursing homes.[4] Therefore long term (direct and indirect) costs are likely to be determined by the number of patients with long term disability.

It follows that stroke unit care will be more cost effective than conventional care if it reduces long term disability without increasing either the length of stay in a hospital or institution or the cost of an episode of inpatient care.

Table 5.1 Proportion of direct costs due to different aspects of hospital care

Aspect of care	Proportion of direct costs
Nursing	81%
Hospital overheads	14%
Investigation	2%
Therapy	1.6%
Medical care	1%
Drugs	0·5%

Adapted from Warlow et al.[3]

Identifying potential costs and benefit

Cost effectiveness analysis

We wished to carry out a cost effectiveness analysis by identifying the costs and benefits associated with stroke units and comparing them with those of conventional care in general medical wards. Ideally this analysis should be performed from a societal perspective, considering all the costs and benefits stemming from a switch to stroke units from conventional care in general wards, but this is inevitably limited by the gaps in the available data.

For the purposes of an economic evaluation which simply aims to compare two models of care, we can exclude the costs and outcomes which are common to both types of care (cost of heating, lighting, food, drugs, etc.). The areas which are likely to differ between stroke units and general medical wards are listed in Table 5.2. A simple qualitative comparison would suggest that if stroke unit care is more cost effective the added benefit would need to be greater than the potential additional costs.

Potential benefits

We have reliable data indicating that stroke unit care has added benefit resulting in more patients surviving, regaining independence, and returning home (Meta-analysis of the stroke unit trials, Chapter 4). The scale of this potential gain in terms of absolute numbers of patients who benefit is outlined in Table 4.2.

Potential costs

Hospital costs
We have presented indirect information suggesting that stroke

Table 5.2   Potential costs and benefits of stroke unit care compared with conventional care in general medical wards

Potential benefits	Potential costs
More patients survive	Staffing of unit (? minor increase)
More patients regain independence	Increased investigation and treatment costs (? minor increase)
More patients return home/fewer need nursing home care	More intensive rehabilitation input (? minor increase)
	Increased bed days in hospital
	Increased use of community services

units may incur slightly higher treatment and investigation costs (Table 3.2). This also suggests that more therapy staff may have been available in some stroke units but probably not more nursing staff (Table 3.2). Nurse staffing costs are one of the main determinants of the costs of inpatient care (Table 5.1).

Length of stay

Data were available for 18 randomised trials; ten trials reported a shorter length of stay in the stroke unit group and eight a more prolonged stay.[5] A pooled analysis[5] looking at the weighted mean difference (Coping with different types of outcome, Chapter 4, p 36) suggested that there was a relative reduction in length of stay in the stroke unit group of 8% (95% CI 3–13%). When calculated in absolute values (days) there was a non-significant reduction of 0.3 days (95% CI to 1.8–1.1 days). We are limited in the extent to which general conclusions can be inferred because trials defined length of stay differently and there was considerable heterogeneity in these results (i.e. more variation than would be expected by chance). However, it seems reasonable to conclude that within the randomised trials stroke unit care did not increase length of stay and may have reduced it.

Costs of care after return home

Patients who return home may require services such as home helps, community nursing, aids, and appliances. In addition, there may be indirect costs for carers who lose productive activity as a result of the patient returning home. We have no data on these costs within the randomised trials and can only make informed guesses.

Measuring costs and benefits

For every 100 patients managed in an organised inpatient (stroke unit) care setting, we can calculate how many extra would enjoy a beneficial outcome or avoid a poor outcome and what the cost implications of these changes would be. Table 4.2 contains absolute outcome data from the stroke unit trials to which we have added local information from a typical British teaching hospital (Table 5.3) on the average length of stay of four patient groups: those who died, were discharged to institutional care, were discharged home physically dependent (see Box 4.2) or were discharged home physically independent. The final column shows the calculated change in numbers of bed days for a cohort of 100 patients treated in a stroke unit as compared to a general medical ward, with a net effect of a reduction of 26 bed days across the different outcome groups.

It is important to recognise that this analysis includes several assumptions.

1. Stroke unit care does not change length of stay for stroke patients in general or for particular subgroups of patients – the first appears to be correct (Potential benefits, above). We also have some unpublished subgroup information from five trials[6-10] which indicates that the average lengths of stay were very similar between the stroke unit and general ward settings for patients who died, who returned home, or who were discharged to an institution.

2. The length of stay data are reasonable and representative; the absolute values for length of stay available from the trials frequently reflected practices in the 1970s and 1980s. We have chosen to use routine hospital data to reflect more closely the current situation (at least in the United Kingdom). Had we used trial data, the absolute length of stay estimates and hence the apparent benefits of stroke unit care would be considerably greater than those presented here. Therefore, our analysis is probably a conservative estimate of the benefit of stroke units.

3. The benefits of stroke unit care apply to all stroke patients. Most trials selected patients to some extent but units which accepted most or all stroke patients[9-12] appeared to be at least as effective at improving patient outcomes and reducing length of stay as those with more selective admission policies.[8,13,14]

4. All stroke patients incur the same (daily) hospital costs. Although not strictly correct (Forbes and Dennis, Scottish Office Report, 1995), this is a reasonable assumption since the main determinants of inpatient costs are nursing costs and overheads (Table 5.1). Therefore the observed variation in costs will relate closely to length of stay in hospital, which we have taken into account.

5. Our estimates are precise. Although our estimates are based on trials data on 2770 patients randomised (Table 5.3), the estimates for each outcome group have wide confidence intervals. They remain the most reliable data available at present.

Economic interpretation of results

Economic "balance sheet"

How can these results be summarised to assist decision makers? From a societal economic perspective (ignoring the fact that different agencies will often bear the costs of hospital, nursing home, and domiciliary care), one option is preferred to another if it has greater benefits and lower costs. Stroke units appear to have a clear advantage over general medical wards in improving disability-free survival but the balance of costs is less clearcut. In our analysis (Table 5.3) the "balance sheet" for a cohort of 100 patients treated in a stroke unit rather than a general medical ward is as follows.

26 less bed days used (assuming no difference in length of stay)
1 fewer patient discharged to institutional care
5 additional patients discharged home

The main issue, therefore, is whether the value of any extra resources used in the stroke unit or in providing home care will exceed the value of resources released. The average Scottish mainland hospital cost per general medical bed day is £192 (*Scottish Health Service Costs, Year ended 31st March 1996,* Information and Statistics Division, Trinity Park House, Edinburgh). The average cost of a nursing home place per week in Scotland is £377 (based on costs updated to 1997 from *Scottish Health Service Costs,* as above). This implies that the value of the resources released is £4992 (192 × 26) in the acute hospital. The value of resources freed in institutional care is £19,604 (377 × 52 × 1) per year. This suggests that, in treating 100 patients, stroke unit care can free resources to the value of £25,596 (£4992 + £19,604) in the first year. This will exceed the value of the extra resources consumed so long as both of the following conditions hold.

1. Any additional hospital costs did not exceed £25,596 per 100 stroke patients (£256 per patient). This seems likely since we have no suggestion of increased nursing staff levels within stroke units and length of stay is likely to be unchanged or reduced (Potential benefits, p 59).
2. The five extra patients discharged home each cost less than £5059 per year. This seems likely since the majority of these patients were independent and so would normally require only

Table 5.3   Analysis of outcomes in stroke units and general wards

Outcome	Percentage of those admitted with each outcome			Average length of stay in hospital (LOS) in days	Change (95% CI) in inpatient bed days per 100 patients (ND×LOS)
	Stroke unit (% of SU patients)	General ward (% of GMW patients)	Net difference (ND) and 95% CI between SU and GMW		
Dead	23	28	−4(−7 to 0)	19	−76(−133 to 0)
Discharged to institutional care	20	22	−1(−4 to +1)	90	−90(−360 to +90)
Discharged to home, physically dependent	18	16	0(−4 to +3)	27	0(−108 to +81)
Discharged home independent	39	33	5(+1 to +8)	28	140(+28 to +224)
				Total	−26

The two left hand columns show the proportion (%) of patients in the stroke unit (SU) and general medical ward (GMW) groups who were in each outcome category at the end of scheduled follow-up (median one year). The middle column shows the net difference (ND) in outcomes (95% confidence interval) per 100 patients treated calculated from the risk difference (Table 4.2). The risk difference takes into account the heterogeneity of the primary trials and so differs slightly from the simple subtraction of the GMW from the SU results. Length of stay (LOS) data are derived from a routine hospital survey. The terms "independent" and "dependent" are described in Box 4.2. Adapted from Table 4.2.

intermittent home care (home help) support and possibly some aids and appliances which cost a fraction of institutional care.

Factors missing from the analysis

We should mention that several factors are missing from this analysis.

- Set-up costs such as training in stroke care or multidisciplinary rehabilitation. These are likely to be relatively modest (Table 3.2), particularly as frequently all that is required is a reorganisation of staff who already have appropriate skills but need a stroke unit to deliver a co-ordinated service.
- Additional indirect effects in the form of losses of production and social benefits. These are likely to be small in this predominantly elderly group.[4]
- Costs to families and to informal carers. Relatives who provide support at home for stroke victims may sustain direct (e.g. aids, home care) and indirect (e.g. loss of earnings) costs.
- Long term costs. We have not established that the benefits of stroke unit care are maintained in the long term and that adverse outcomes are not simply delayed. One of the trials (Trondheim) has reported preliminary data from a prolonged follow-up of patients (Indredavik *et al*, Presentation to the 8th Nordic Meeting on Cerebrovascular Diseases, Trondheim, 1995) indicating that the early benefits of stroke unit care, and presumably the cost reductions, are sustained for at least five years.
- Sensitivity analysis. Ideally, we should include repeated analyses which examine the influence of "best case" and "worst case" scenarios on our conclusions. For example, we could look at the influence of altering hospital and nursing home costs or of reducing the estimate of the number of patients who benefit. We have presented the average estimates of benefit and cost.

Even if these missing factors do make stroke units more expensive, the additional resources consumed can be set against the improvements in outcomes following stroke. Thus, even in a "worst case" scenario stroke units seem likely to be more cost effective than general medical wards.

Implications of the analysis

In the least favourable analysis stroke unit care achieves better patient outcomes for a modest increase in costs; at best, it releases health care resources. However, the costs included here are economic costs relating to the value of resources used and freed; they are not the same as financial costs. For example, there will be no saving of money if the bed days released are simply taken up by increased demand from other areas of a health service. There is a further problem that resources released may not easily be moved between budgets. While the impact of stroke units may be efficient from a societal perspective, the distribution of costs and resources freed is important. The extra burden may fall on community services (such as social work and general practice) whereas the resources freed are in acute hospitals and nursing homes.

There are many limitations which prevent this being a conclusive economic evaluation. In particular, we have had to rely on a mix of outcome data from randomised trials and data derived from our own services. Large clinical trials and systematic reviews are increasingly required to demonstrate the effectiveness of interventions (Chapter 2). Economic evaluation of such studies would be greatly improved if good quality economic data were collected specifically for inclusion in meaningful analyses.

6: Implications for planning stroke services

This systematic review provides convincing evidence for the effectiveness of stroke units but little specific data to guide the organisation of one's own service. We have addressed this problem by first drawing on our own experience of co-ordinating stroke services and then by asking some trialists to tell us how they do things. We are therefore drawing on practical experience and common sense as well as the evidence to produce a more complete account of how to organise inpatient stroke care.

Evidence based stroke care

This systematic review indicates that any nihilism which surrounds stroke care is unjustified and that better organisation of inpatient stroke care improves patient outcomes (Chapter 4) and is probably cost effective (Chapter 5). In this penultimate chapter we have tried to fill the gap between the evidence available (in randomised trials) and the practical everyday decisions which we have to make on the organisation of our service. We have tried to be explicit about the level of evidence we are using (Levels of evidence, Chapter 2, p 8) and, wherever possible, to base our decisions on evidence from randomised trials (level I). Our practical guide is based on:

- the systematic review outlined in the preceding chapters (level I);
- four case studies of "typical" stroke units which contributed to the systematic review (level III) – they provide a more detailed account of stroke unit procedures and practices (Appendix). They were chosen because they:
  - were representative of the two most common approaches to stroke unit care;
  - were recently evaluated in a randomised trial;
  - showed evidence of effectiveness in their own right;
- other published information (levels I–III), with some indication

of the methodological quality of that information;
• the authors' personal experience and anecdote (level IV).

Comprehensive stroke services

The term "stroke service" is a broad one[1] and should incorporate the range of facilities required to provide comprehensive care for stroke (Figure 6.1). Important functions include provision of a prompt and accurate diagnosis and assessment of patients' problems, appropriate acute medical and surgical treatment, appropriate rehabilitation including discharge planning for those admitted to hospital, initiation of secondary prevention measures, and follow-up to prevent and identify late problems. Certain facilities (Box 6.1) aid the delivery of various components of a

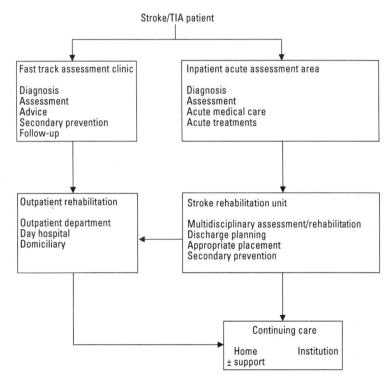

Figure 6.1 Comprehensive stroke service. Outline of a comprehensive stroke service including both inpatient and outpatient care in the acute and rehabilitation phases of the illness. (Modified from Dennis and Langhorne.[1])

Box 6.1   Facilities within a comprehensive stroke service

- Neurovascular clinic for prompt assessment and initiation of secondary prevention for outpatients
- Inpatient facilities for acute medical care and multidisciplinary rehabilitation
- Continuing care and support facilities for severely dependent patients
- Close links with primary care, social services, and the voluntary sector

---

comprehensive stroke service. It is clear that stroke units form only one part of a comprehensive stroke service although this is likely to be a very important part, particularly in regions where the majority of stroke patients are admitted to hospital.[2]

What kind of stroke unit?

This question can be broken down into several parts.

Stroke patients only or mixed rehabilitation service?

Should the unit manage only stroke patients or attempt to deliver an organised system of stroke care within a generic disability service? We would suggest that stroke-specific units should be the preferred model of care, particularly in hospitals which manage large numbers of stroke patients. Not only have disease-specific units been more widely studied in randomised trials, they also tended to achieve better outcomes (What general policies should be applied? Chapter 4, p 51, level I) and allow for more specialisation among team members (Table 3.3, level III), which may be an advantage. In circumstances where this is not practical, for example hospitals which manage only a few stroke patients, many of the benefits of stroke unit care are available within a mixed disability setting such as a geriatric rehabilitation ward or rehabilitation medicine unit.

Stroke ward or mobile stroke team?

Mobile teams can deliver stroke unit-type care to patients scattered across a variety of wards. However, we believe that geographically defined stroke units are the current preferred option but that mobile stroke teams could be further evaluated in trials. Although our broad definition of a stroke unit (Defining the intervention, Chapter 3, p 20) has allowed the inclusion of both geographically defined stroke wards and mobile stroke teams, only one randomised trial focused specifically on a mobile team and it did not produce definitive results in its own right ([3], level I). The bulk of the evidence about the effectiveness of stroke units has therefore come from trials of geographically defined stroke units (Table 3.1, level I). We also have experience of both types of service and have found that an important advantage of having patients in one place is that nursing staff can play a greater part in the rehabilitation process (level IV). Co-ordinating the care of patients scattered across a variety of wards is difficult and stroke patients managed in acute areas have to compete for nursing time with others who are perceived as having more urgent needs (for example, chest pain). Potentially important aspects of rehabilitation such as regular toileting to maintain continence and dignity may be seen as having a lesser priority when nursing resources are limited. Geographically defined stroke units remove this competition for nursing time and may allow the nurses to take on a new role as facilitators of patients' independence and providers of continued therapy over the full 24-hour period (level IV). Stroke units can also provide a focus for the development of research, fundraising and volunteer support groups and make it easier to introduce and monitor the adherence to clinical guidelines and protocols (level IV). In practice, geographically defined units often overspill during busy periods and the stroke unit staff have to operate as a mobile team to some patients housed outwith their ward.

Acute or rehabilitation unit?

Currently there is little evidence to support units which intervene only in the acute period. Whatever model is adopted, it must be able to provide care for many weeks if required (What general policies should be applied?, Chapter 4, p 51, level I). Units employing either acute or delayed admission (both of which then offered several weeks of care) both appeared to improve outcomes over that of general medical wards. However, we cannot say whether either approach was superior since the case mix differed and there have been no direct comparisons between these two models of unit. Admitting all patients with stroke directly into a unit allows the introduction of a standardised approach with assessment and treatment protocols (Table 3.4, level III) and may result in earlier involvement of paramedical staff (Table 3.4, level III). It also facilitates research and probably allows skills to be focused (level IV). In our experience the acute care needs of some stroke patients may often be more appropriately met within an acute ward than on one where the emphasis is on rehabilitation (level IV). For example, very sick patients might require care that would disrupt a rehabilitation unit at a time when they are unlikely to benefit from a rehabilitative environment. However, at least three examples of a stroke unit ([4-6], level I) have operated such a system which combines acute care and rehabilitation. An alternative pragmatic approach, which draws on both personal experience and some information from randomised trials (Table 3.1), is that patients might be admitted to an acute assessment area, either within a medical ward or as part of an acute stroke unit, and then move to a stroke rehabilitation unit as soon as they can benefit from that environment. One potential disadvantage of this model is the apparent lack of continuity of care but this can be reduced by ensuring that the stroke unit team work beyond the confines of the rehabilitation ward and participate closely in the patient's care from the time of admission to hospital.

Staffing a stroke unit

This area can be broken down into two parts, namely, which parent department should be responsible for running a stroke unit and what should the staffing structure be?

In which department should the unit be established?

Whoever is responsible for stroke care should have the necessary knowledge, training and, above all, enthusiasm to take on the task (level IV). We base this view on the observation that the stroke units included in this systematic review were run by geriatricians, neurologists, general physicians, and specialists in rehabilitation medicine and appeared to achieve similar benefit (What general policies should be applied?, Chapter 4, p 51, level I). Indeed, a more striking feature was the similarity of systems of care developed in units which were housed in different departmental settings (Characteristics of different models of stroke unit, Chapter 3, p 29, level III). The most appropriate professional group to run stroke care will vary from place to place and no single group may be equipped to provide all aspects of care (level IV). For example, in the United Kingdom most stroke patients are managed by general physicians and geriatricians. British neurologists may have the knowledge and training to diagnose and investigate stroke but most do not have the time, facilities or training in rehabilitation to run the stroke service alone. In the UK geriatricians are often in the best position to take a leading role although most would need some extra training in neurology and support from neurologists when dealing with younger patients and unusual causes of stroke. Ideally the development of stroke units and stroke services in general would draw upon the skills of different individuals to help deliver the best quality care to patients (level IV).

What staff are needed?

Stroke units require medical, nursing, physiotherapy, occupational therapy, speech and language therapy, and social work input as a basic minimum; almost all the units in the systematic review included these staff (Table 3.2, level III). Other disciplines (Box 6.2) have an important role in selected patients (level IV).

The question of the most appropriate staffing levels cannot be fully answered here. Trialists did not usually report staffing levels and when we could obtain these, they were defined and calculated

---

Box 6.2   Stroke team staff

Core team	Physician
	Nurses
	Physiotherapists
	Occupational therapists
	Speech and language therapists
	Social worker
Other professionals who may have a role in the management of a stroke patient	Audiologist
	Chaplain
	Chiropodist
	Clinical psychologist
	Dentist
	Dietician
	Neurosurgeon
	Psychiatrist
	Pharmacist
	Ophthalmologist
	Radiologist
	Rheumatologist
	Vascular surgeon

in different ways with different degrees of cross-cover from other departments. Therefore staffing levels are difficult to equate across different trials, but we have summarised the range of estimates for a hypothetical ten-bed stroke unit (Appendix, level III):

- *medical* – consultant medical input of 0.5–1 whole-time equivalents (WTE) per ten patients;
- *medical* – junior medical staffing input of 0.4–0.8 WTE per ten patients;
- *nursing* input of 7–12 WTE per ten patients (this includes a mixture of skill levels);
- *physiotherapy* of 1–2 WTE per ten patients;
- *occupational therapy* of 0.9–1.3 WTE per ten patients;
- *speech and language therapy* of 0.2–0.6 WTE per ten patients;
- *social work* input of < 0.4–0.7 WTE per ten patients.

These levels are broadly in line with our own personal experience of staffing in such units[1] but we must emphasise that such estimates should be considered only a rough guide.

Stroke unit policies

This broad category includes the size of the stroke unit, patient selection policies, and duration of patient stay.

Stroke unit size

Most of the stroke units within the systematic review were of moderate size (6–15 beds) although some mixed rehabilitation units were as large as 30 beds (unpublished data). In our experience (level IV) the co-ordination of multidisciplinary care becomes practically difficult once the number of beds begins to exceed 15. Therefore in larger hospitals there may be a case for splitting larger wards into two, each with their own administrative structure. The total number of beds required might theoretically be calculated from the age- and sex-specific stroke incidence, details of the hospital catchment population and referral patterns, and hospital activity data ([7], level III). Unfortunately the numbers of admissions will not be constant around the year and pressure on the stroke unit will fluctuate, usually being heavier in the winter.[7] For instance, one survey in a general hospital in Edinburgh[1] which has a 15-bed stroke unit and admits between 200 and 250 stroke patients each year found that the number of patients with stroke in the hospital on any one day varied between nine and 35. Therefore, whatever the organisation, it must be able to cope with such fluctuations.

One problem of the geographically defined stroke ward is the inevitable limit on spaces. This may be overcome by ensuring the stroke unit is part of a larger area and that the multidisciplinary team can extend their care to patients unable to be admitted to a stroke ward (level IV). Ideally, most patients would be in a rehabilitation area rather than an acute general ward. This requires fluctuations of staffing as well as beds so that members of the team can call on other specialist colleagues when necessary. Inevitably, there may be times when resources are not adequate to meet all the demands of the patients, at which point the team may have to make difficult decisions on prioritising input (level IV). The multidisciplinary team can provide a supportive environment for its members in these stressful circumstances.

Patient selection criteria

There appears to be a good case (Which patients benefit?, Chapter 4, p 48, level I) for offering stroke unit care to a wide range of patients, extending at least from those who have mild disability initially (e.g. requiring assistance with walking) through to those with severe strokes (e.g. no sitting balance). Our systematic review provides little information to guide the care of patients with very minor stroke or transient ischaemic attacks (many of whom can be managed out of hospital) and those in coma. There do not appear to be any grounds for excluding patients on the basis of age. Sometimes alternative services, such as age-related geriatric rehabilitation services, are available which could offer some of the benefits of stroke unit care (What general policies should be applied?, Chapter 4, p 51, level I). The best solution might be to seek a local agreement based on the needs of individual patients whereby older patients with multifactorial problems are managed within the geriatric medical services and those with purely stroke problems are managed within a disease-specific stroke unit (level IV).

Duration of stay

Some of the units in this review set a maximum length of stay. The only real rationale for this is to allow the management of resources and to prevent blocking of beds. If the unit is of sufficient size for the population needs, works flexibly, and is efficient in discharging patients, then a defined maximum length of stay should not be required (level IV). It has been argued that patients who are no longer improving but have to wait for placement elsewhere should not be kept in a stroke unit. However, the unit may offer the best environment to maintain any functional improvement which has been gained. Moving patients may be detrimental and can compromise continuity of care (level IV). Moves under these circumstances should be considered only when beds are limited and patients who will gain more from the unit environment are waiting to be admitted (level IV).

Practices and procedures

So far we have focused on general aspects of stroke unit structure and policy. However, it seems likely that many benefits of stroke units result from the policies and procedures applied in day to day practice. For the purposes of discussion we have split these into communication, care pathways, and education. We would suggest that those developing units should aim to conform with the practices commonly described in the trials.

Communication: Multidisciplinary team

All stroke units should have a formal multidisciplinary team meeting at least once per week, probably lasting between one and three hours which is chaired by a senior staff member (a senior physician in the trials reviewed) (Table 3.2, level I). These meetings are not routinely attended by patients or carers. The meeting introduces the patients to the multidisciplinary team and provides a forum for multidisciplinary assessment and problem identification, setting of short and long term rehabilitation goals, and decision making (Appendix, level III). Some units include a few minutes set aside for education (level IV).

In addition to the formal multidisciplinary team meeting, some units hold more frequent, less formal meetings usually attended by nursing and therapy staff (Appendix, level III) at which patients and carers may be present (see Communication: carers, below). In addition, informal daily communication on the wards is probably important (Appendix, level III). In our experience (level IV) several interlinking systems of communication are required to ensure that good multidisciplinary working can develop without requiring team members to spend too much of their time in meetings.

Communication: Carers

A distinctive feature of the stroke units in our systematic review was the early, active involvement of carers in the rehabilitation process (Table 3.2, level I). Stroke unit staff should actively attempt to make contact with patients, relatives, and carers within one week of their admission (Appendix, level III). Although carers are not usually invited to the formal multidisciplinary team meetings, they may be invited to the informal meetings with nursing and therapy staff and to rehabilitation sessions in the ward or gym (Appendix, level III). Carers may be involved in care for patients when in the unit, which may provide training in the skills they will need later and help give some insight into what caring for the patient will entail (level IV). Patients and carers should routinely be provided with information on stroke disease, stroke management, secondary prevention, and support services. Potentially useful approaches include information boards, books available on loan, and the hosting of carers support groups (Appendix, level III).

Care pathways

Although there were some significant variations in the management pathways of individual patients in the stroke unit case studies (Appendix), there were many similarities.

Assessment

The medical assessment includes a history and examination to establish the neurological impairment, plus routine blood biochemistry and haematology, and a cranial computed tomography scan (Appendix, level III). Other investigations such as carotid artery Doppler ultrasound assessment, echocardiography, and magnetic resonance imaging are used in selected patients (Appendix, level III).

The nursing assessment (Appendix, level III) includes the general care needs of the patient, including a formal scoring of pressure score risk and an assessment of swallowing (in three of the case studies swallowing assessment was carried out by nursing staff and in one by speech and language therapy staff).

The initial assessment by therapy staff includes an evaluation of the patient's impairments and disabilities (Appendix, level III).

Management
Medical

The systematic review cannot reliably guide specific medical

75

therapies. We now have much more reliable, direct information from large randomised trials to support the routine use of aspirin[8,9] but not heparin.[8] There were a range of medical practices reported from the four case studies, reflecting to some extent the difference in emphasis between acute and rehabilitation care. The use of intravenous fluids, heparin for severe hemiparesis, aspirin, and antipyretics were reported in individual case studies (Appendix, level III). The early use of antibiotics for suspected infections was a more consistent feature (Appendix, level III). Thrombolytic agents such as streptokinase and tissue plasminogen activator did not feature within the stroke unit trials. However, if these agents become established as effective therapies then acute stroke units will be needed to ensure their safe use (level IV).

Nursing

The nursing management includes attention to the patient's general care needs, maintaining the patient in a correct posture and position, and regular observation of key characteristics such as airway, swallowing, nutritional status, continence, and skin integrity (Appendix, level III). The nurses also have a key role as a link between therapy staff and patients by incorporating good quality movement and handling into daily practice (Appendix, level III). Observational studies from the Nottingham unit ([10], level III) indicated that patients within the stroke unit were more likely to have active contact with nursing and therapy staff, were more active during their routine day, and were more likely to be in a good body position than control patients managed in a general ward.

Therapy input

Therapy input should begin early (Appendix, level III). Within the case studies physiotherapy was routinely commenced within 24 hours of admission to the unit (or on the next working day) while the onset of occupational therapy assessment and treatment ranged from less than 24 hours to three days. There are no randomised trials which have provided reliable evidence concerning the optimum type, timing or intensity of therapy input.[11] In the case studies, the specific therapy technique did not appear to be important since no single therapy approach was used for either physiotherapy or occupational therapy; movement science, Bobath, a modified individualised form of Bobath, Carr and Shepherd, and proprioceptive neuromuscular facilitation approachs were all used (Appendix, level III). Physiotherapy input ranged from 30–60 minutes per day while occupational therapy d from 20–40 minutes per day (Appendix, level III).

No single monitoring scale was used consistently across units (Appendix, level III) but several scales were used including TELER,[12] Barthel index,[13] Frenchay Activities Index,[13] Rivermead,[13] and the Scandinavian Stroke Scale.[13]

Prevention of complications

Standardised formal protocols should be used to detect dysphagia and prevent aspiration, and the routine use of intravenous fluids or nasogastric supplements considered in any case of impaired swallowing (Appendix, level III). There also appears to be an important role for supervised feeding and careful positioning during feeding (Appendix, level III).

Prophylaxis for deep venous thrombosis should be guided by large clinical trials. We now know that the routine use of heparin can prevent deep venous thrombosis but is associated with an increase in intracranial haemorrhage and confers no overall clinical benefit.[8] The routine use of compression stockings has not been evaluated in stroke patients but is effective in high risk medical and surgical patients[14] and would appear to be the current choice. Compression stockings were the most commonly used intervention in the case studies but two units also used subcutaneous heparin in high risk patients. Early mobilisation and careful positioning and turning are used to prevent both deep venous thrombosis and other problems of immobility (Appendix, level III).

The risk of infection was reduced through the avoidance of urinary catheters where possible, careful positioning and turning, early mobilisation, and the aggressive and early treatment of suspected infections (Appendix, level III).

Discharge planning

Early contact should be made with carers and patients to make appropriate assessments regarding eventual discharge (Appendix, level III). Not all of the units in the case studies could arrange a predischarge home visit although in our experience this can be very useful (level IV). In one unit (Orpington) discharge plans began as soon as it became apparent that the patient would be able to manage toileting, transfers, and communication. In this case a joint home visit was made by a social worker and a member of the multidisciplinary team. The role of liaison nurse follow-up is currently unclear[15,16] and the subject of further trials. This was available in two of the case study units (Perth, Nottingham). The

two acute admission units (Perth, Trondheim) referred selecte
patients on to rehabilitation services outwith the unit

Education, training, and beliefs

A programme of education and training appears to be an important feature of stroke unit care (Table 3.2, level I). Education and training for the members of the multidisciplinary team involved in the case studies comprised informal weekly education events and a programme of formal education ranging from one to six days per year (Appendix, level III). These teams were asked what they believed were the important characteristics of an effective stroke unit. The most consistent themes were:

- co-ordinated multidisciplinary team care involving integration of patient, carer, and multidisciplinary team input;
- early and intensive rehabilitation;
- having staff with an interest in stroke care;
- active involvement of carers in the process of rehabilitation.

Other less consistently reported views were having a programme of research and aggressive early use of intravenous fluids and antipyretic medication.

Overcoming resistance to change

Although there is now good evidence for the effectiveness of organised inpatient (stroke unit) care, such developments are often resisted by professional colleagues who perceive them as a threat. One argument is that they will inevitably consume more resources and increase the cost of inpatient care. The main benefits of stroke unit care are probably derived from improved organisation and teamwork, rather than extra staff or facilities. Our economic analysis (Chapter 5) indicates that stroke units are unlikely to consume extra resources and may even release them for use elsewhere. In particular, they are unlikely to increase length of stay in hospital and may reduce it ([17], Potential costs, Chapter 5). As patients seem to have a better functional status on discharge from stroke units, hospital resources do not appear to be saved simply at the expense of community resources and families, where they are less easily measured. One circumstance where the establishment of a stroke unit may increase staff costs is in hospitals which have inadequate nursing or paramedical staff numbers to provide a basic rehabilitation service, in which case it is not the stroke unit which is at fault but the inadequacies of the previous service (level IV).

Professional colleagues may fear that stroke units will divert resources from their own specialty but this seems unlikely if they allow a more efficient use of existing resources (especially beds) which may eventually release resources for use by other specialties (Chapter 5). They may worry that a specialist stroke team will reduce the skills of their junior medical, nursing, and paramedical staff and reduce their access to patients for teaching undergraduates. However, this can be easily overcome by rotating staff and students through the unit (level IV).

Opposition may be reduced by adopting an evolutionary approach (level IV), perhaps beginning with the introduction of assessment protocols before establishing an assessment area or stroke team working in general medical wards. This can then provide the basis for the establishment of a geographically defined stroke unit. Where resistance continues, it is important to bear in mind that purchasers of medical services are generally keen to purchase services where there is scientific evidence of effectiveness and which relate to important medical problems. Within the UK, stroke is a *Health of the Nation* target[18] and so should be seen as a priority for future action. However, the type of stroke service adopted needs to be flexible as its structure will be influenced by local conditions such as needs, resources, geography, personnel, and politics (level IV).

7: Implications for future research

There are many outstanding questions concerning the organisation of inpatient stroke care, the provision of alternatives to inpatient care, and how best to provide rehabilitation services for those who have returned home. Fortunately, a number of randomised trials are currently under way which address these areas, with plans for a systematic review evaluation of these and previous relevant trials. Hopefully, a more systematic and objective approach to evaluating new service developments[1] will avoid some of the difficulties which have hampered the interpretation of the stroke unit trials and delayed their widespread implementation.

Current state of knowledge

The preceding chapters have summarised the evidence supporting organised inpatient (stroke unit) care. However, we have also tried to indicate the limitations of these analyses and, in particular, to point out the areas where it is difficult to make confident practical inferences. What can we confidently conclude about the organisation of stroke care and what are the outstanding questions and uncertainties?

- The only components of a comprehensive stroke service (Box 6.1) which have been subject to a large number of randomised trials concern the organisation of inpatient care.
- Organised inpatient stroke care, which fulfils the broad definition of a multidisciplinary stroke unit, can achieve better patient outcomes than conventional care in general medical wards.
- Both disease-specific (dedicated stroke units) and generic disability services (mixed assessment/rehabilitation units) appear to achieve better results than conventional care in general medical wards, but we do not know which of these two former approaches is more effective or efficient.
- A number of specific models of stroke unit care have been tested in randomised trials; both those combining acute care with

rehabilitation and those focusing only on post-acute rehabilitation were more effective than conventional care in general medical wards.

- We can identify some general features which are characteristic of an effective stroke unit but we cannot be confident about which specific features are important.

Outstanding questions

Bearing in mind what has been outlined above, we would suggest that some of the key outstanding questions are as follows.

Can acute stroke units (intervening only in the first few days after stroke) bring about additional improvements in patient outcomes? Acute units almost certainly facilitate early assessment and the delivery of acute medical treatment and research but the impact of these functions on patient outcomes remains unclear. As only one randomised trial of an acute stroke unit has been completed, (Table 3.1) we currently have very limited evidence to answer this question.

Can a generic disability service (mixed assessment and rehabilitation ward) achieve similar outcomes to a disease-specific dedicated stroke ward? This question is of practical interest because it could dictate whether services dedicated to stroke care should be developed widely or whether stroke patients are managed within a mixed disability setting.

Can mobile stroke teams (which do not have a ward base but provide multidisciplinary care to patients housed in a number of wards) achieve similar outcomes to a dedicated stroke ward? To some extent, this is a less interesting question because the mobile stroke team is likely to incur the same basic costs as one based within a dedicated ward and there are major practical limitations to this model of care (Stroke ward or mobile stroke team?, Chapter 6, p 68).

Can community based services prevent admission of patients to hospital? There is considerable interest within the United Kingdom in community based services which aim to prevent patients being admitted to hospital and to provide all support and care within the home environment. These are variously termed "home care services" or "hospital at home". Much of the enthusiasm for this type of service derives from a belief among health care purchasers that they will reduce costs and be more popular with patients and carers. To date, only one controlled, but not randomised, trial[2] has evaluated this model of care in stroke. This study, which was based in Bristol, England, evaluated the impact of a multidisiciplinary home care team being offered to general practitioners in half the health care districts within the city and was compared with the conventional practice in the other half of the city. There was a trend towards slightly better patient outcomes with the home care team although these were not statistically significant. However, the home care team did not prevent admissions to hospital; there was almost identical hospital bed use in the two groups. Therefore, as the home care team incurred an additional cost over the conventional services, the overall health care costs were increased by this model of care. Further trials of hospital at home for acute patients are currently under way.[3]

Can domiciliary services accelerate discharge home for hospitalised stroke patients? This is another area of current interest partly because of the political drive towards reducing the number of hospital beds and partly because it is perceived to offer a form of care which is both cheaper and preferable to stroke patients and carers. At present, this model of care should be considered experimental and is currently the subject of several randomised trials. Ideally, these trials should compare their early supported discharge service with what we now believe to be the current gold standard, i.e. organised inpatient (stroke unit) care.

What outpatient rehabilitation should be routinely provided after discharge from hospital? This really incorporates a number of questions regarding the provision of outpatient rehabilitation including out patient physiotherapy, occupational therapy, liaison nursing, social work, and counselling interventions. At present, there is considerable variation in the provision of such services which presumably reflects uncertainty about their relative benefits and costs. A number of randomised trials have examined or are currently examining these questions.

What is the best setting for providing outpatient rehabilitation? This has conventionally involved comparisons between the hospital based care (often in a day hospital) and home based (domiciliary) care. Two substantial randomised controlled trials[4,5] have compared hospital based and domiciliary rehabilitation after stroke but a combined analysis of these two trials[6] concluded that there was insufficient statistical power to demonstrate any difference in outcomes between these two forms of service. Further trials comparing these two forms of care are currently under way.

What are the important components of the "black box" of organised inpatient (stroke unit) care? All the previous trials have examined a complex intervention containing many interrelated components. We will only be confident about the effectiveness of individual interventions if they are each subjected to reliable randomised trials. Recent large trials have established a role for the routine use of aspirin in ischaemic stroke[7,8] and concluded that routine heparin use is not indicated.[7] Many questions remain, such as the best policies for providing nutritional support, best positioning of patients, routine use of antipyretic medication, optimal control of blood pressure and blood glucose level, and the optimal type, intensity, and duration of therapy input.

In conclusion, this systematic review of organised inpatient (stroke unit) care can be considered a first step; further randomised trials will be required if we are to evaluate and implement truly evidence based comprehensive stroke services. Planned prospective collaboration in the development of these trials[1] would avoid many of the problems encountered in the development and evaluation of stroke unit care and would greatly aid their subsequent interpretation.

Appendix: Descriptions of stroke unit care

In this appendix we provide some additional information about four of the stroke units which were tested within randomised trials. These examples were chosen because:

- they represented two common models of stroke unit; a combined acute/rehabilitation stroke unit and a rehabilitation stroke unit;
- they were evaluated in a recent randomised trial, so that the trialists could give a good account of practices during the trial;
- they represented a spread of three different countries and departmental settings;
- the trials all indicated some benefit in reducing disability or handicap.

We collected information using standard qualitative research methods[1] including a structured interview followed by a detailed questionnaire and two patient case studies ("vignettes"). This does not represent a true systematic review approach but a systematic survey of four selected examples. They are intended to describe some of the practices and procedures which took place within the stroke unit trials. However, it is important to appreciate some methodological limitations:

- information is based on what trialists believed was happening (we did not confirm this with direct observation);
- the questionnaires usually used an open question format (e.g. "What procedures were used to prevent complications?") in order to avoid directing responses in a particular way. A consequence of this is that some of the apparent differences between units may reflect what the trialist believed was important to report rather than what was actually done. Responses to these open questions have been highlighted with an asterisk*;
- the information on staffing levels cannot be reliably compared between units because of different definitions of tasks, different levels of cross-cover and different staffing structures (What staff are needed?, Chapter 6, p 71).

The authors of the individual stroke unit examples should be cited as indicated in Table 8.1.

Table 8.1 General details of stroke units

Unit	Authors	Size (no. of beds)	Type of unit	Parent department	General*
Perth[2]	Hankey Chan Deleo Ancliffe Grille Stewart-Wynne	12	Combined acute and rehabilitation	Neurology	Established in the major city teaching hospital in Perth, Western Australia, through a joint initiative between neurology and general medicine. Stroke beds established within a 21-bed neurology ward
Trondheim[3]	Indredavik Bakke Solberg Rokseth Haahein Holme Nilsen Schjolberg	6	Combined acute and rehabilitation	General medicine	Established in the main city hospital of Trondheim, Norway, serving population of 200,000
Orpington[4]	Kalra	13	Rehabilitation	Geriatric medicine	Established in an urban general hospital to provide rehabilitation for hospitalised stroke patients
Nottingham[5]	Berman Edmans Foster Goodwin Grant O'Reilly Stout	15	Rehabilitation	Geriatric medicine	Established in an urban teaching hospital within the city of Nottingham to provide rehabilitation for patients admitted to hospital

Table 8.2 Staffing of stroke units

Unit	Medical*	Nursing* (during 24-hour period)	Physiotherapy*	Occupational therapy*	Speech and language therapy*	Other*
Perth	Cross-cover arrangement with 2 neurologists and 3 general physicians. 1·0 WTE registrar and resident	6–7 WTE trained staff. 1–3 WTE care assistants. Various specialist interests. NB: Describes the staff numbers for 12 stroke beds only	1·2 WTE therapists (all grades)	0·6 WTE senior therapist. 0·5 WTE junior therapist (more than in general wards)	0·75 WTE therapists	Input from one social worker (shared with neurology) Dietician Pharmacist
Trondheim	Consultant physician with interest in stroke/ rehabilitation. Junior medical cross-cover	Slightly greater than conventional nursing complement	1·0 WTE therapist	Conventional OT input	Conventional SLT input	No routine social worker input
Orpington	0·2 WTE consultant grade (general and geriatric medicine with interest in stroke). 0·5 WTE senior house officer (general medical experience)	6·5 WTE trained staff. 6·0 WTE untrained staff (specialist interest in rehab)	1·5 WTE therapists (all grades)	1·5 WTE therapists (all grades)	0·3 WTE therapists (all grades)	Social worker allocated to unit
Notingham	Approximately 0·3 WTE consultant geriatrician (with interests in stroke and rehabilitation). 0·6 WTE junior medical cover	10·5 WTE trained staff (specialist interest in stroke unit rehabilitation). 7·7 WTE untrained staff	3 WTE therapists (all grades)	2 WTE therapists (all grades)	One therapist (also had other responsibilities outside stroke unit)	Clinical psychology (0·5 WTE). Social work (0·6 WTE)

Key: WTE, whole time equivalent; OT, occupational therapy; SLT, speech and language therapy

Table 8.3 Admission and discharge policies of stroke units

Unit	Patient criteria*	Proportion (%) of all stroke patients	Average (maximum) delay before admission*	Average (maximum) time in unit*	Discharge arrangements*
Perth	Any acute stroke patients (provided bed available in the unit)	40–50% of patients referred to hospital	<1 day (7 days)	25 days (unlimited)	Most suitable surviving patients referred for further specialist rehabilitation. Liaison nurse follow-up
Trondheim	Acute stroke patients (excluding coma, resident in nursing home, resident in distant district, symptoms of more than 1 week)	70–80% of patients referred to hospital	16 hours (7 days)	16 days (42 days)	A minority of patients move to specialist rehabilitation facility
Orpington	Hospitalised patient requiring rehabilitation at 2 weeks after stroke	65% of patients admitted to hospital	14 days	35 days (unlimited)	Usually to final placement (home or institution)
Nottingham	Hospitalised patients (excluding reduced consciousness, unstable medical condition, previous severe disability, unable to transfer with 2 persons)	17% of patients admitted to hospital	14 days (30 days)	76 days (unlimited)	Usually to final placement (home or institution). Liaison nurse follow-up

Table 8.4 Communication within stroke units

| Unit | Multidisciplinary communication | | | Communication with relatives/carers | |
	Formal meetings	Informal meetings*	Other*	Formal meetings	Other*
Perth	1 per week (1 hour) chaired by consultant. Report assessments, set goals, report on progress, future plans (5 mins teaching integrated into the meeting)	Regular "family meeting" with carers, nursing, medical, PT, OT, SLT, SW staff and stroke liaison nurse	Informal contact in unit on a daily basis	No routine attendance	See "Informal meetings". Carers routinely contacted during first week and invited to attend rehabilitation sessions
Trondheim	1 per week (1–2 h) chaired by consultant. Report assessments, set goals, discuss problems, discharge planning	2–3 per week involving nursing, therapy staff, and often patients and carers	Informal communication in unit on a daily basis	No routine attendance	Carers routinely contacted and invited to become involved in rehabilitation and to attend informal meetings
Orpington	1 per week (2½ h) chaired by consultant. Report assessments, progress, set goals, discuss problems, make decisions	1 per week (1–2 h). Nursing, PT, OT, SLT, SW staff meeting	Daily communication on unit	No routine attendance	Carers routinely contacted and invited to attend rehabilitation sessions
Nottingham	1 per week (2 h) usually chaired by consultant. Report on progress, goals and discharge planning	1 per week. Nurses, PT, OT, SLT and clinical psychology staff	Daily communication within unit	No routine attendance	Multidisciplinary family case conferences arranged. Routinely involved in rehabilitation sessions

Key: PT, physiotherapy; OT, occupational therapy; SLT, speech and language therapy; SW, social work

Table 8.5   Routine assessment procedures

Unit	Medical*	Nursing*	Therapy*	Other*
Perth	History and examination. Routine biochemistry and haematology, ECG, CXR, CT scanning. Selective use of other investigations (MRI, carotid Doppler, echo)	Clinical history. Vital signs. Fluid balance. Airway, swallowing, continence, skin integrity (Norton score), nutritional assessment (on admission to unit)	Gowland recovery score. Berg-Alan scale. TELER. Barthel index. Upper limb tests and others	Swallowing and speech assessment by SLT staff
Trondheim	History and examination. Routine biochemistry and haematology, ECG, CXR, CT scanning, selective use of other investigations	Clinical history. Vital signs. Fluid balance. Systematic observation (own observation score). Swallowing assessment. Scandinavian Stroke Scale	Assessment of impairments and disabilities (Barthel index) (within 24 h of admission)	
Orpington	History and examination. Routine biochemistry and haematology, ECG, CXR, CT scanning. Selective use of other investigations	Clinical history, vital signs. Standardised swallowing and nutrition assessment. Continence, skin integrity. Oral hygiene. Discharge assessment	Functional assessment of impairments. ADL charting. Aphasia screening test	
Nottingham	History and examination. Routine biochemistry, haematology, ECG, CXR, CT scanning. Selective use of echocardiography and carotid Doppler	Clinical history. Routine observation/monitoring. Nutrition score. Pressure sore risk. Barthel ADL Index	Rivermead motor assessment. Indicator of physical progress following stroke. Rivermead ADL score (within 24 h)	Clinical psychology assessments. Speech therapy. Swallowing assessment

Key: CT, computed tomography; MRI, magnetic resonance imaging; ECG, electrocardiograph; CXR, chest X-ray; ADL, activities of daily living

Table 8.6   Routine management procedures

Unit	Medical*	Nursing*	Physiotherapy*	Occupational therapy*	Speech and language therapy*	Other*
Perth	Assessment of cause. Secondary prevention. Selective use of anticoagulants. Avoid acute blood pressure reduction. Prevent complications	Careful positioning and handling. Bowel and bladder care. Food and fluid balance. Pressure area care	Bobath. Proprioceptive neuromuscular facilitation (PNF). Carr and Shepherd approaches (30–60 min per day; 5 days per week)	Cognitive and perceptual retraining. Bobath, PNF, Brumstrom approaches (40 mins per day; 5 days per week)	Monitoring with Royal Brisbane Dysphagia Outcome Scale. Communication skills retraining	
Trondheim	Regular use of intravenous fluids. Low dose heparin for severe hemiparesis. Antipyretic medication. Oxygen if drowsy. Antibiotics if aspiration suspected	Careful positioning and handling. Food and fluid balance. Active stimulation, mobilisation and ADL training	Movement science approach. Early active mobilisaton (30 mins per day; 5 days per week)	Functional approach (OT involvement with approximately 50% of patients)	Management of swallowing and communication problems	
Orpington	Routine aspirin use. Selective heparin use. Avoid aggressive BP reduction. Avoid complications	Careful positioning and handling. Bowel and bladder care. Pressure area care. Informal therapy support. Discharge planning	Functionally orientated care (30–60 mins per day; 5 days per week)	Functionally orientated care (30 mins per day; 5 days per week)	Regular monitoring of swallowing and communication problems	Social work assessment within 1 week
Nottingham	Antithrombotic secondary prevention measures. Complications treated. Avoid aggressive BP reduction	Positioning and handling. Pressure area care. Bowel and bladder care (see Prevention of complications)	Variety of approaches (Bobath, Carr and Shepherd) (45–60 mins per day; 5 days per week)	Variety of approaches (usually Bobath) (45–60 mins per day; 5 days per week)	Regular monitoring of dysphagia. Functional approach to communication problems	Clincal psychology (50% of patients). Social work input (most patients)

Key: BP, blood pressure; OT, occupational therapy

Table 8.7 Strategies for prevention of complications

Unit	Aspiration*	Dehydration/malnutrition*	Venous thromboembolism*	Contractures*	Pressure sores*	Urinary tract infection*
Perth	Clinical swallowing assessment. Positioning. Modified feeding	Identify high risk patients. Dietary supplementation. Tube feeding (NG, PEG) as required	Graduated compression stockings. Selective heparin use	Positioning, stretching, selective use of muscle relaxant drugs	Identify high risk patients. Regular turning. Continence care. Selective use of pressure cushions	Avoid unnecessary catheterisations (bladder US to assess residual volume). Avoid constipation/dehydration
Trondheim	Clinical swallowing assessments. Careful positioning (antibiotics if aspiration suspected)	Nasogastric feeding and/or intravenous fluids for patients with swallowing problems	Early active mobilisation. Low dose heparin for severe hemiparesis	Careful positioning. Early active mobilisation	Regular turning, early active mobilisation	Avoid unnecessary catheterisation
Orpington	Positioning. Patient and carer education. Modified diets. Supervised feeding	Close monitoring of food and fluid balance	Passive and active exercises. Selective use of heparin	Passive exercises. Positioning and support	Regular turning. Skin care. Continence care. Selective use of pressure mattresses and cushions	Avoid unnecessary catheterisation. Personal hygiene. Fluid balance
Nottingham	Optimal positioning. Supervision and monitoring of feeding. Modified diets	Supplementary intravenous fluids or tube feeding if required. Food supplements if no swallowing problems	Regular, early mobilisation. Anti-embolic stockings	Careful positioning, moving and handling. Passive mobilisation. Occasional splint or Baclofen use	Identify high risk patients. Regular repositioning. Selective use of pressure mattresses and cushions	Avoid dehydration and unnecessary catheterisation. Cranberry juice

Key: NG, nasogastric; PEG, percutaneous endoscopic gastrostomy; US, ultrasound investigation

Table 8.8   Education, training, and audit

Unit	Format of education/training*	Monitoring of service quality*	Information to patients and carers*
Perth	6 workshops per year for nurses. 6 workshops per year for therapists. Regular education at multidisciplinary meetings. Weekly 30-min stroke unit seminar	Regular audit. Patient and staff questionnaires	Regular discussion. Leaflets. Education board. Stroke information sessions
Trondheim	Regular seminars in stroke care. Induction programme for new staff	Regular audit and data collection (stroke data bank)	Regular discussion and advice. Stroke information materials provided
Orpington	2-day multidisciplinary course twice per year (lectures and practical sessions). Weekly multidisciplinary tutorials	Regular audit and data collection	Stroke information. General health advice. Advice on benefits and support. Training in disability management
Nottingham	Weekly seminars in multidisciplinary stroke care. Therapist teaching sessions every 2 weeks. Induction programme for new staff	Regular audit and survey of patient satisfaction. Feedback from stroke support group	Stroke Association booklets. Stroke unit booklet. Presentations to relatives. Support group

Table 8.9   Attitudes regarding stroke unit effectiveness

Unit	What are the effective components of stroke unit care?*
Perth	Multidisciplinary team approach (regular weekly meetings). Standardised procedure in meetings co-ordinated by team leader. Education of staff, patients, and families. Staff interest in stroke care. Research programme
Trondheim	The development of a team approach. Early intensive rehabilitation programme. Involvement of relatives in the rehabilitation process. Liberal use of intravenous fluids to prevent dehydration and anti-pyretic medication to reduce fever. Education and training of staff, patients, and relatives
Orpington	Good interdisciplinary co-ordination. Specialist nature of the unit. Goal setting and monitoring objectives. Partnership with patients and families. Education and training of staff, patients, and families. Regular audit
Nottingham	Co-ordinated multidisciplinary care. Nursing integration with the rehabilitation team. Improved nursing care and education. Complete rehabilitation philosophy. More thorough and co-ordinated discharge planning. Specialist expertise of staff

92

Glossary of terms

Absolute outcomes Results (outcomes) of a trial expressed as the absolute number of patients with that outcome. (see also relative outcomes).

Acute stroke unit See stroke unit.

Applicability See external validity.

Attrition bias Systematic error (bias) due to systematic differences in the withdrawal of patients from the treatment and control groups (See Chapter 2 for example).

Bias Systematic error producing results that differ from the true value. (See p 10 for example).

Blinding Ensuring that the participants and/or investigators in a trial are not aware of which treatment the participant was getting. Drug studies are often 'double blind' where neither the participant nor investigator knows their treatment. Rehabilitation trials are usually 'single blind' because the participant is aware of the treatment they have received.

Case series Study based on a series of cases (patients) with the condition of interest.

Case mix The mix of important characteristics (eg. age, social class, stroke severity) within a patient group. Randomisation should produce a very similar case mix in the intervention and control groups.

Clinical heterogeneity Dissimilarities between the trials included in a review in terms of the participants, context/settings, treatments/interventions (see also heterogeneity, statistical heterogeneity).

Combined acute/rehabilitation stroke unit see stroke unit.

Computer generated randomisation A random sequence, generated by computer, for allocating participants in a trial to intervention and control groups (see also Random allocation).

Confidence interval The range within which the true size of effect of a treatment is likely to lie. For example the 95% confidence interval includes the true value in 95% of cases.

Continuous outcome An outcome measure (eg. height) expressed on a continuous scale (see also dichotomous outcome).

Cost benefit An economic analysis comparing the returns on investing resources in services designed to treat different health problems.

Cost effective An economic analysis comparing the cost of different ways of tackling the same health problem (eg. stroke unit versus general wards) in terms of the number of beneficial outcomes achieved divided by financial cost.

Dedicated stroke unit See stroke unit.

Detection bias Systematic error (bias) due to systematic differences in the way outcomes are assessed. This can be overcome by 'blinding' the outcome assessment (See p 12 for example).

Dichotomous outcome An outcome in binary form (eg. dead or alive).

Direct comparison Comparison within a trial where patients are randomised to one of two (or more) competing forms of care (see indirect comparison).

Direct cost Cost (eg. drugs, nursing care) which is directly attributable to a treatment or service (see indirect cost).

Disability Any restriction or lack of ability to perform activity within the range considered normal for a human being.

Effectiveness The extent to which a treatment, procedure or service does people more good than harm.

Efficacy The extent to which a treatment, procedure or service improves the outcome for people under ideal cicumstances.

Error The degree to which a result differs from the 'true' value. This can be random or systematic (bias).

External validity (syn applicability, generalisability)
The degree to which the results of an observation hold true in other settings, particularly routine health care situations (see Chapter 3).

Generalisability See external validity.

Haemorrhagic stroke Stroke caused by bleeding from blood vessels in the brain (see also ischaemic stroke).

Handicap A disadvantage for a given individual resulting from an impairment or disability that limits or prevents the fulfilment of a role that is normal for that individual.

Healthcare intervention Broad term for any treatment, procedure or service intended to improve the health of the recipient.

Heterogeneity Dissimilarity between trials included in a systematic review such that the participants, treatments/interventions and endpoints are not comparable. Significant heterogenity may mean that combining trial results into a single summary statistic is unwise. The opposite of heterogeneity is homogeneity. (See also clinical heterogeneity, statistical heterogeneity).

Historical controls   A comparison group taken from an earlier period of time before an intervention was used (an unreliable comparison group).

Indirect cost   Cost (eg. loss of earnings) indirectly attributable to an illness or treatment (see Direct cost).

Indirect comparison   Where two (or more) interventions are compared against an independent control group rather than each other. Much less reliable than a direct comparison (see above) for establishing which intervention is more effective.

Intention-to-treat   In an intention-to-treat analysis all the participants in a trial are analysed according to the treatments/ intervention that they were originally meant to get regardless of whether they actually received it. All patients are included in the primary analysis even if they have died or dropped out of the trial. These analyses are favoured in assessments of effectiveness as they minimise bias and mirror more closely the performance of a treatment in normal practice.

Internal validity   The degree to which the results of a study are likely to be true. Randomised controlled trials which have minimised the risk of bias have high internal validity.

Intervention study   A trial in which a treatment/intervention is evaluated by allocating patients to either the intervention or an alternative(s) and then recording their outcomes. Encompasses randomised controlled trials and controlled clinical trials. (See also observational study).

Ischaemic stroke   Stroke caused by occlusion of a blood vessel resulting in (ischaemic) brain damage.

Meta-analysis   A statistical technique which summarises the results of several studies into a single estimate giving greater weight to results from larger studies

Mixed assessment/ rehabilitation unit   See stroke unit.

Multidisciplinary   Practices involving more than one healthcare discipline. In stroke rehabilitation this usually involves at least medical, nursing, physiotherapy, occupational therapy, speech and language therapy, and social work staff.

Number needed to treat (NNT)   One measure of the magnitude of treatment/intervention effectiveness; the number of people who would need to receive a specific treatment to prevent one specific outcome. It is calculated as 100% divided by (% treatment patients with outcome - % control patients with outcome).

Observational study   Study which observes the outcomes in patients who may or may not be exposed to a particular treatment/intervention. It differs from an intervention study in that no attempt is made to allocate patients to a particular treatment group. Observational studies are too prone to bias to provide a reliable indication of treatment effectiveness.

Odds ratio   The ratio of the chances (odds) that an outcome (event) will happen in the treatment group to the 'odds' that the event will happen in the control group, ie

No of treatment patients experiencing an event	No of control patients experiencing an event
divided by	
No of treatment patients not experiencing an event	No of control patients not experiencing an event

If the odds ratio is 1 then the effect of the treatment is no different from control. If the odds ratio is <1 then the event was less common in the treatment group. Odds ratios are usually expressed together with their confidence interval (see confidence interval).

Outcomes   Specified results within a trial (eg death, disability score).

Performance bias   Systematic differences in the care received by treatment and control patients in addition to the aspect of care under study. This is difficult to eliminate in complex health service or rehabilitation trials (see p 11).

Publication bias   A major problem in reviewing research because studies with 'positive' results are more likely to be published and therefore are easier to trace. Treatments/interventions that have produced neutral or 'negative' results in trials are more likely to remain unpublished. Systematic reviews which fail to include unpublished trials may therefore conclude that the treatment/intervention is more effective than is truely the case (see p 17).

Quality of life   Subjective measure based on the patient's perceived outcome. Comparable to handicap.

Quasi–Random   Methods of prospective allocation of participants to treatment or control groups which may produce balanced groups but are not strictly random (and therefore subject to selection bias). Examples of quasi-random allocation include day of the week, bed availability, alternation.

Random error   Error which is governed by chance; in contrast to bias which is a systematic error.

Random allocation   Method used to conceal the random sequence from the individuals who are entering participants into a trial. Random allocation implies that each participant in the trial has an equal chance of receiving each of the possible treatments/interventions. Examples include the use of sequentially numbered opaque sealed envelopes. (see also Computer generated randomisation)

Randomised controlled trial (RCT)   A trial where individuals (or other experimental units) followed up in the study were assigned prospectively to one of two (or more) forms of healthcare using random allocation

Relative outcome   The outcomes of patients receiving a treatment/intervention in relation to the outcomes in control patients. Examples include the % reduction in outcome event, odds ratio and relative risk. Results expressed as relative outcomes often appear more impressive than those expressed as absolute outcomes eg Aspirin may cause a 20% reduction in deaths (relative outcome) which equates to a drop from 5% of patients dying to 4% (absolute outcomes).

Rehabilitation stroke unit   See stroke unit.

Risk difference   A measure of the difference in the absolute risk of an adverse outcome occurring in the intervention group as opposed to the controls (ie. % risk in intervention group − % risk in controls). See also absolute outcomes.

Secondary prevention   Treatments given to prevent the recurrence of an illness. In the present context it refers to treatments given to people who have suffered a stroke or transient ischaemic attack to prevent recurrent stroke or other vascular event.

Selection bias   The introduction of bias in a trial through systematic differences in the selection of participants for the treatment/intervention and control groups. This is probably the main source of bias in health services research and can be minimised by random allocation of patients to treatment and control groups.

Statistical heterogeneity   The degree of dissimilarity between the results of individual trials within a meta-analysis. Statistical tests are used to determine if differences between trials could be due solely to chance (random error) or if they indicate the

trials are measuring different effects. Significant statistical heterge-
neity indicates that the combining of trial results into a single
summary analysis may be unwise.

Statistical power   A measure of a trial's ability to detect a
clinically important difference based on the number of participants
who are entered and the random variability of the outcomes
measured. Many trials do not include enough patients to answer
the question of effectiveness.

Statistical significance   All trial results are subject to the play
of chance. The p-value from statistical tests indicate how likely it is
that the trial results are just chance findings. Significance is the
level at which we decide to take something seriously (1 in 20 = 5%,
1 in 100 = 1%). 95% confidence intervals which impinge on 1
indicate a result which is not statistically significant.

Stroke   Focal neurological cerebral deficit caused by vascular
disease.

Stroke unit   A number of definitions of stroke unit have been
used in the past. Most definitions allude to hospital-based stroke
care designed to improve the outcome of stroke patients. Tradition-
ally this has been defined by the co-ordinated multidisicipinary
team care these patients receive. This definition can include the
following:

1 Stroke ward   a geographically defined area where stroke
   patients receive stroke unit care.
2 Stroke team   a mobile team delivering stroke unit care to
   patients in a variety of wards.
3 Dedicated stroke unit   a disease-specific stroke unit managing only stroke patients.
4 Mixed assessment/rehabilitation unit   a generic disability
   unit (which fulfils the definition of a stroke unit) specialising in
   the management of disabling illnesses including stroke.
5 Acute stroke unit   a stroke unit accepting patients acutely
   and continuing for several days (usually < 1 week).
6 Combined acute/rehabilitation stroke unit   a stroke unit
   accepting patients acutely but continuing care for several
   weeks if necessary.
7 Rehabilitation stroke unit   a stroke unit accepting patients
   after a delay of 1-2 weeks and continuing care for several seeks
   if necessary.

Subarachnoid haemorrhage   A type of stroke in which there
is bleeding into the subarachnoid space around the brain. These
patients were usually excluded from stroke unit studies because

early neurosurgical treatment is often required.

Subdural haematoma   A condition which can mimic stroke caused by a blood clot on the surface of the brain. These patients were usually excluded from stroke unit studies because early neurosurgical treatment is often required.

Systematic review   A review in which evidence (usually from randomised controlled trials) on a topic has been systematically identified, appraised, and summarised according to predetermined critera. Such reviews can be systematic (taking steps to reduce bias) without using statistical synthesis (meta-analysis) to reduce imprecision.

Transient ischaemic attack (TIA)   Focal neurological symptoms caused by cerebrovascular disease which resolve within 24 hours.

Validity   The degree to which any result (of a measurement, study, trial) is likely to be true and free of systematic error (bias). See also internal validity, external validity.

References

Preface

1. Warlow CP, Dennis MS, van Gijn J *et al. Stroke: a practical guide to management.* Edinburgh: Blackwell Science, 1996.
2. King's Fund Consensus Conference. Treatment of stroke. *Br Med J* 1988;**297**:128.
3. The Cochrane Library [database on disk and CD-ROM]. Update software, 1996.

Chapter 1

1. Murray CJL, Lopez AD. Mortality by cause for eight regions of the world: global burden of disease study. *Lancet* 1997;**349**:1269.
2. Sudlow CLM, Warlow CP. Comparing stroke incidence worldwide: what makes studies comparable? *Stroke* 1996;**27**:550–8.
3. Bamford J, Sandercock P, Dennis M, Burn J, Warlow C. Classification and natural history of clinically identifiable subtypes of cerebral infarction. *Lancet* 1991;**337**:1521–6.
4. Langton Hewer R. Rehabilitation after stroke. *Q J Med* 1990;**76**:659–74.
5. Isard PA, Forbes JF. The cost of stroke to the National Health Service in Scotland. *Cerebrovasc Dis* 1992;**2**:47–50.
6. Evers SMAA, Engel GL, Ament AJHA. Cost of stroke in the Netherlands from a societal perspective. *Stroke* 1997;**28**:1375–81.
7. Bergman L, van der Meulen JHP, Limburg M, Habbema JDF. Costs of medical care after first-ever stroke in the Netherlands. *Stroke* 1995;**26**:1830–6.
8. Adams GF. Prognosis and prospect of strokes. In: Anonymous. *Cerebrovascular disability and the ageing brain.* Edinburgh: Churchill Livingstone, 1974.
9. Waylonis GW, Keith MW, Aseff JN. Stroke rehabilitation in a midwestern county. *Arch Physical Med Rehab* 1973;**54**:151–5.
10. Peacock PB, Riley CHP, Lampton TD, Raffel SS, Walker JS. The Birmingham stroke, epidemiology and rehabilitation study. In: Stewart GT. Ed. *Trends in epidemiology.* Springfield, IL: CC Thomas, 1972.
11. Dow RS, Dick HL, Crowell FA. Failures and successes in a stroke program. *Stroke* 1974;**5**:40–7.
12. Bonner CD. Stroke units in community hospitals: a how-to guide. *Geriatrics* 1973;**28**:166–70.
13. Garraway WM. Stroke rehabilitation units: concepts, evaluation and unresolved issues. *Stroke* 1985;**16**:178–81.
14. McCann C, Cuthbertson RA. Comparison of two systems for stroke rehabilitation in a general hospital. *J Am Geriatr Soc* 1976;**24**:211–16.
15. Feigenson JS, Gitlow HS, Greenberg SD. The disability orientated rehabilitation unit – a major factor influencing stroke outcome. *Stroke* 1979;**10**:5–8.
16. Ebrahim S. *Clinical epidemiology of stroke.* Oxford: Oxford University Press, 1990.
17. Isaacs B. Five years experience of stroke unit. *Health Bull (Edinburgh)* 1977;**35**:93–8.

18. Norris JW, Hachinski VC. Intensive care management of stroke patients. *Stroke* 1976;7:573–6.
19. Kennedy FB, Pozen TJ, Gableman EH, Tuthill JE, Zaentz SD. Stroke intensive care – an appraisal. *Am Heart J* 1970;80:188–96.
20. Drake WE, Hamilton MJ, Carlsson M, Kand F, Blumenkrantz J. Acute stroke management and patient outcome: the value of neurovascular care units (NCU). *Stroke* 1973;4:933–45.
21. Pitner SE, Mance CJ. An evaluation of stroke intensive care: results in a municipal hospital. *Stroke* 1973;4:737–41.
22. Garraway WM, Akhtar AJ, Hockey L, Prescott RJ. Management of acute stroke in the elderly: preliminary results of a controlled trial. *Br Med J* 1980;280:1040–4.
23. Strand T, Asplund K, Eriksson S, Hagg E, Lithner F, Wester PO. A non-intensive stroke unit reduces functional disability and the need for long-term hospitalisation. *Stroke* 1985;16:29–34.
24. Von Arbin M, Britton M, de Faive U *et al*. A study of stroke patients treated in a non-intensive stroke unit or in general medical wards. *Acta Med Scand* 1980;208:81–5.
25. Stevens RS, Ambler NR, Warren MD. A randomised controlled trial of a stroke rehabilitation ward. *Age Ageing* 1984;13:65–75.
26. Sivenius J, Pyorala K, Heinonen OP, Salonen JT, Riekkinen P. The significance of intensity of rehabilitation after stroke – a controlled trial. *Stroke* 1985;16:928–31.
27. Wood-Dauphinee S, Shapiro S, Bass E. A randomised trial of team care following stroke. *Stroke* 1984;5:864–72.
28. Stone SP. The Mount Vernon stroke service: a feasibility study to determine whether it is possible to apply the principles of stroke management to patients and their families on general medical wards. *Age Ageing* 1987;16:81–8.
29. Anonymous. Report of Geriatric Committee Working Group on strokes. London: Royal College of Physicians, 1974.
30. King's Fund Consensus Conference. Treatment of stroke. *Br Med J* 1988;297:128.
31. Lindley RI, Amayo EO, Marshall J, Sandercock PAG, Dennis M, Warlow CP. Hospital services for patients with acute stroke in the UK: the Stroke Association Survey of Consultant opinion. *Age Ageing* 1995;24:525–32.
32. Steggmayr B, for the Steering Committee for "Riks-Stroke". A national registry for quality assessment of acute stroke care in Sweden. *Cerebrovasc Dis* 1997;7 (suppl 4): 69 abstract.
33. Sackett D, Rosenberg W, Richardson S *et al*. *How to practise and teach evidence based medicine*. Edinburgh: Churchill Livingstone, 1996.
34. Feldman DJ, Lee PR, Untertrecker J *et al*. A comparison of functionally oriented medical care and formal rehabilitation in the management of patients with hemiplegia due to cerebrovascular disease. *J Chron Dis* 1962;15:297–310.
35. Indredavik B, Bakke F, Solberg R *et al*. Benefit of stroke unit: a randomised controlled trial. *Stroke* 1991;22:1026–31.
36. Ilmavirta M, Frey H, Erila T, Fogelholm R. Does treatment in a non-intensive care stroke unit improve the outcome of ischaemic stroke? Det 7 Nordiska Motet om Cerebrovasculara Sjukdomar, Jyvaskyla, Finland 1993.
37. Langhorne P, Williams BO, Gilchrist W, Howie K. Do stroke units save lives? *Lancet* 1993;342:395–8.
38. WHO Regional Office for Europe, European Stroke Council, European Federation of Neurological Societies, International Stroke Society, World Confederation for Physical Therapy, World Federation of Occupational Therapists, Pan European Consensus Meeting on Stroke Management, 1996.
39. Stroke Unit Trialists' Collaboration. A collaborative systematic review of the

randomised trials of organised inpatient (stroke unit) care after stroke. *Br Med J* 1997;**314**:1151–9.

Chapter 2

1. US Department of Health and Human Services. Agency for Health Care Policy and Research. Acute pain management: operative or medical procedures and trauma. AHCPR 92–0023 Rockville, MD: AHCPR, 1993.
2. Davenport RJ, Dennis MS, Warlow CP. Effect of correcting outcome data for case mix: an example from stroke medicine. *Br Med J* 1996;**312**:1503–5.
3. Mulrow CD, Oxman AD. *Cochrane Collaboration Handbook*. In: The Cochrane Library [database on disk and CD-ROM]. 1996.
4. Murray CJL, Lopez AD. Mortality by cause for eight regions of the world: global burden of disease study. *Lancet* 1997;**349**:1269.
5. Ottenbacher KJ, Jannell S. The results of clinical trials in stroke rehabilitation research. *Arch Neurol* 1993;**50**:37–44.
6. Campbell MJ, Julious SA, Altman DG. Estimating sample sizes for binary, ordered categorical, and continuous outcomes in two group comparisons. *Br Med J* 1995;**311**:1145.
7. International Stroke Trial Collaborative Group. The International Stroke Trial (IST): a randomised trial of aspirin, subcutaneous heparin, both, or neither among 19435 patients with acute ischaemic stroke. *Lancet* 1997;**349**:1569–81.
8. CAST (Chinese Acute Stroke Trial) Collaborative Group. CAST: randomised placebo-controlled trial of early aspirin use in 20000 patients with acute ischaemic stroke. *Lancet* 1997;**349**:1641–9.
9. European Cartoid Surgery Trial Collaborative Group. MRC Cartoid Surgery Trial: interim results for patients with severe (70–99%) or with mild (0–30%) cartoid sterosis. *Lancet* 1989;**1**:175–80.
10. Gladman J, Barer D, Langhorne P. Specialist rehabilitation after stroke. Effective in the short term, but more work needed in the long term. *Br Med J* 1996;**312**:1623–24.
11. O'Connor GT, Buring JE, Yusuf S *et al.* An overview of randomized trials of rehabilitation with exercise after myocardial infarction. *Circulation* 1989;**80**:234–44.
12. Oldridge NB, Guyatt GH, Fischer ME, Rimm AA. Cardiac rehabilitation after myocardial infarction. *JAMA* 1988;**260**:945–50.
13. Mulrow CD. The medical review article: state of the science. *Ann Intern Med* 1987;**106**:485.
14. Mulrow CD. Rationale for systematic reviews. *Br Med J* 1994;**309**:597–9.
15. Antiplatelet Trialists' Collaboration. Collaborative overview of randomised trials of antiplatelet therapy. I: Prevention of death, myocardial infarction and stroke by prolonged antiplatelet therapy in various categories of patients. *Br Med J* 1994;**308**:81–106.
16. Chalmers TC, Frank CS, Reitman D. Minimizing the three stages of publication bias. *JAMA* 1990;**263**:1392–5.
17. Dickersin K, Min YI. NIH clinical trials and publication bias. *Online J Curr Clin Trials* April 1993.
18. Shultz KF, Chalmers I, Grimes DA *et al.* Assessing the quality of randomisation from reports of controlled trials published in obstetrics and gynaecology reports. *JAMA* 1994;**272**:125–8.
19. Gotzsche PC. Methodology and overt and hidden bias in reports of 196 double-blind trials of nonsteroidal antiinflammatory drugs in rheumatoid arthritis. *Controlled Clin Trials* 1989;**10**:31.
20. Thompson SG. Why sources of heterogeneity in meta-analysis should be investigated. *Br Med J* 1994;**309**:1351–5.

Chapter 3

1. Mulrow CD, Oxman AD. *Cochrane Collaboration Handbook*. In: The Cochrane Library [database on disk and CD-ROM]. 1996.
2. Garraway WM. Stroke rehabilitation units: concepts, evaluation and unresolved issues. *Stroke* 1985;**16**:178–81.
3. Bonner CD. Stroke units in community hospitals: a how-to guide. *Geriatrics* 1973;**28**:166–70.
4. Bonita R. Epidemiology of stroke. *Lancet* 1992;**339**:342–4.
5. The Cochrane Library [database on disk and CD-ROM]. Update software, 1996.
6. Stroke Unit Trialists' Collaboration. A collaborative systematic review of the randomised trials of organised inpatient (stroke unit) care after stroke. *Br Med J* 1997;**314**:1151–59.
7. Stewart LA, Parmar MKB. Meta-analysis of the literature or of individual patient data: is there a difference? *Lancet* 1993;**341**:418–22.
8. Peacock P, Riley C, Lampton T, Raffel S, Walker J. The Birmingham stroke, epidemiology and rehabilitation study. In: Stewart G. Ed. *Trends in epidemiology.* Springfield, IL: Thomas C C, 1972.
9. Stevens RS, Ambler NR, Warren MD. A randomised controlled trial of a stroke rehabilitation ward. *Age Ageing* 1984;**13**:65–75.
10. Garraway WM, Akhtar AJ, Hockey L, Prescott RJ. Management of acute stroke in the elderly: follow up of a controlled trial. *Br Med J* 1980;**281**:827–9.
11. Fagerberg B, Blomstrand C. Do stroke units save lives? [letter]. *Lancet* 1993;**342**:992.
12. Kaste M, Palomaki H, Sarna S. Where and how should elderly stroke patients be treated? A randomized trial. *Stroke* 1995;**26**:249–53.
13. Gordon EE, Kohn KH. Evaluation of rehabilitation methods in the hemiplegic patient. *J Chron Dis* 1966;**19**:3–16.
14. Sivenius J, Pyorala K, Heinonen OP, Salonen JT, Riekkinen P. The significance of intensity of rehabilitation after stroke – a controlled trial. *Stroke* 1985;**16**:928–31.
15. Wood-Dauphinee S, Shapiro S, Bass E. A randomised trial of team care following stroke. *Stroke* 1984;**5**:864–72.
16. Feldman DJ, Lee PR, Unterecker J *et al.* A comparison of functionally orientated medical care and formal rehabilitation in the management of patients with hemiplegia due to cerebrovascular disease. *J Chron Dis* 1962;**15**:297–310.
17. Aitken PD, Rodgers H, French JM, Bates D, James OFW. General medical or geriatric unit care for acute stroke? A controlled trial. *Age Ageing* 1993;**22** (suppl 2):4–5.
18. Juby LC, Lincoln NB, Berman P. The effect of a stroke rehabilitation unit on functional and psychological outcome. A randomised controlled trial. *Cerebrovasc Dis* 1996;**6**:106–10.
19. Kalra L, Dale P, Crome P. Improving stroke rehabilitation: a controlled study. *Stroke* 1993;**24**:1462–7.
20. Kalra L, Eade J. Role of stroke rehabilitation units in managing severe disability after stroke. *Stroke* 1995;**26**:2031–4.
21. Hankey G, Deleo D, Stewart-Wynne EG. Acute hospital care for stroke patients: a randomised trial. *Cerebrovasc Dis* 1995;**5**:228.
22. Ilmavirta M, Frey H, Erila T, Fogelholm R. *Does treatment in a non-intensive care stroke unit improve the outcome of ischaemic stroke?* Jyvaskyla, Finland: Det 7 Nordiska Motet om Cereborvasculara Sjukdomar, 1993.
23. Indredavik B, Bakke F, Solberg R. *et al* Benefit of stroke unit: a randomised controlled trial. *Stroke* 1991;**22**:1026–31.
24. Strand T, Asplund K, Eriksson *et al.* A non-intensive stroke unit reduces

functional disability and the need for long-term hospitalisation. *Stroke* 1985;**16**:29–34.

25. Hamrin E. Early activation after stroke: does it make a difference? *Scand J Rehab Med* 1982;**14**:101–9.

Chapter 4

1. Antiplatelet Trialists' Collaboration. Collaborative overview of randomised trials of antiplatelet therapy. I: Prevention of death, myocardial infarction and stroke by prolonged antiplatelet therapy in various categories of patients. *Br Med J* 1994;**308**:81–106.
2. Bracken MB. Statistical methods for analysis of effects of treatment in overviews of randomised trials. In: Sinclair JC, Bracken MB. Eds. *Effective care of the newborn infant.* Oxford: Oxford University Press, 1992.
3. Peto R. Why do we need systematic overviews of randomised trials? *Stat Med* 1987;**6**:233–40.
4. Der Simonian R, Laird N. Meta-analysis in clinical trials. *Controlled Clin Trials* 1986;**7**:177–88.
5. Stroke Unit Trialists' Collaboration. A collaborative systematic review of the randomised trials of organised inpatient (stroke unit) care after stroke. *Br Med J* 1997;**314**:1151–9.
6. Bamford J, Sandercock P, Dennis M, Burn J, Warlow C. Classification and natural history of clinically identifiable subtypes of cerebral infarction. *Lancet* 1991;**337**:1521–6.
7. Davenport RJ, Dennis MS, Warlow CP. Effect of correcting outcome data for case mix: an example from stroke medicine. *Br Med J* 1996;**312**:1503–5.
8. Donnan GA. Lifesaving for stroke. *Lancet* 1993;**342**:383–4.
9. Kalra L, Dale P, Crome P. Improving stroke rehabilitation: a controlled study. *Stroke* 1993;**24**:1462–7.
10. Kalra L, Eade J. Role of stroke rehabilitation units in managing severe disability after stroke. *Stroke* 1995;**26**:2031–4.
11. Hankey G, Deleo D, Stewart-Wynne EG. Acute hospital care for stroke patients: a randomised trial. *Cerebrovasc Dis* 1995;**5**:228.
12. Indredavik B, Bakke F, Solberg R *et al.* Benefit of stroke unit: a randomised controlled trial. *Stroke* 1991;**22**:1026–31.
13. Strand T, Asplund K, Eriksson S *et al.* A non-intensive stroke unit reduces functional disability and the need for long-term hospitalisation. *Stroke* 1985;**16**:29–34.
14. Barer D, Gibson P, Ellul J and the GUESS Group. Outcome of hospital care for stroke in 12 centres. *Age Ageing* 1993;**22** (suppl 3):15.
15. Wade D. Measurement in neurological rehabilitation. In: Wade D., Ed. *Activities of daily living (ADL) and extended ADL tests.* Oxford: Oxford University Press, 1992.
16. Kaste M, Palomaki H, Sarna S. Where and how should elderly stroke patients be treated? A randomized trial. *Stroke* 1995;**26**:249–53.
17. Sivenius J, Pyorala K, Heinonen OP, Salonen JT, Riekkinen P. The significance of intensity of rehabilitation after stroke – a controlled trial. *Stroke* 1985;**16**:928–31.
18. Wood-Dauphinee S, Shapiro S, Bass E. A randomised trial of team care following stroke. *Stroke* 1984;**5**:864–72.
19. Juby LC, Lincoln NB, Berman P. The effect of a stroke rehabilitation unit on functional and psychological outcome. A randomised controlled trial. *Cerebrovasc Dis* 1996;**6**:106–10.
20. Sachet DL, Richardson WS, Rosenberg W, Haynes RB. *Evidence-based medicine: How to practice and teach EBM.* New York: Churchill Livingstone, 1997.
21. Garraway WM. Stroke rehabilitation units: concepts, evaluation and unresolved

issues. *Stroke* 1985;**16**:178–81.
22. Davey Smith G, Song F, Sheldon T. Cholesterol lowering and mortality: the importance of considering initial level of risk. *Br Med J* 1993;**306**:1367–73.
23. Peto R, Collins R, Gray R. Large-scale randomized evidence: large, simple trials and overviews of trials. *J Clin Epidemiol* 1995;**48**:23–40.
24. Counsell CE, Clark MJ, Slattery J, Sandercock PAG. The miracle of DICE therapy for acute stroke: fact or fictional product of subgroup analysis? *Br Med J* 1994;**309**:1677–81.
25. Oxman AD, Guyatt GH. A consumer's guide to subgroup analyses. *Ann Intern Med* 1992;**116**:78–84.
26. Stroke Unit Trialists' Collaboration. How do stroke units improve patient outcomes? A collaborative review of the randomised trials. *Stroke* 1997;**28**:2139–44.
27. Mays N, Pope C. *Qualitative research in health care.* London: BMJ Publishing Group, 1996.
28. Ilmavirta M, Frey H, Erila T, Fogelholm R. *Does treatment in a non-intensive care stroke unit improve the outcome of ischemic stroke?* Jyvaskyla, Finland: Det 7 Nordiska Motet om Cereborvasculara Sjukdomar, 1993.
29. Peacock P, Riley C, Lampton T, Raffel S, Walker J. The Birmingham stroke, epidemiology and rehabilitation study. In: Stewart G. Ed. *Trends in epidemiology.* Springfield, IL: Thomas C C, 1972.
30. Stevens RS, Ambler NR, Warren MD. A randomised controlled trial of a stroke rehabilitation ward. *Age Ageing* 1984;**13**:65–75.
31. Gordon EE, Kohn KH. Evaluation of rehabilitation methods in the hemiplegic patient. *J Chron Dis* 1966;**19**:3–16.
32. Feldman DJ, Lee PR, Unterecker J *et al.* A comparison of functionally orientated medical care and formal rehabilitation in the management of patients with hemiplegia due to cerebrovascular disease. *J Chron Dis* 1962;**15**:297–310.
33. Aitken PD, Rodgers H, French JM, Bates D, James OFW. General medical or geriatric unit care for acute stroke? A controlled trial. *Age Ageing* 1993;**22** (suppl 2):4–5.
34. Hamrin E. Early activation after stroke: does it make a difference? *Scand J Rehab Med* 1982;**14**:101–9.
35. Garraway WM, Akhtar AJ, Hockey L, Prescott RJ. Management of acute stroke in the elderly: follow up of a controlled trial. *Br Med J* 1980;**281**:827–9.
36. Lindley RI, Amayo EO, Marshall J, Sandercock PAG, Dennis M, Warlow CP. Hospital services for patients with acute stroke in the UK: the Stroke Association Survey of Consultant opinion. *Age Ageing* 1995;**24**:525–32.
37. Stroke Unit Trialists' Collaboration. A systematic review of specialist multi-disciplinary (stroke unit) care for stroke inpatients. In: Warlow C, van Gijn J, Sandercock P. Eds. *Stroke module of Cochrane Database of Systematic Reviews.* London: BMJ Publishing Group, 1995.

Chapter 5

1. Sachet DL, Richardson WS, Rosenberg W, Haynes RB. *Evidence-based medicine: How to practice and teach EBM.* New York: Churchill Livingstone, 1997.
2. Isard PA, Forbes JF. The cost of stroke to the National Health Service in Scotland. *Cerebrovasc Dis* 1992;**2**:47–50.
3. Warlow CP, Dennis MS, van Gijn J *et al. Stroke: a practical guide to management.* Edinburgh, Blackwell Science, 1996.
4. Evers SMAA, Engel GL, Ament AJHA. Cost of stroke in the Netherlands from a societal perspective. *Stroke* 1997;**28**:1375–81.
5. Stroke Unit Trialists' Collaboration. A collaborative systematic review of the randomised trials of organised inpatient (stroke unit) care after stroke. *Br Med*

J 1997;**314**:1151–9.

6. Garraway WM, Akhtar AJ, Hockey L, Prescott RJ. Management of acute stroke in the elderly: follow up of a controlled trial. *Br Med J* 1980;**281**:827–9.
7. Wood-Dauphinee S, Shapiro S, Bass E. A randomised trial of team care following stroke. *Stroke* 1984;**5**:864–72.
8. Juby LC, Lincoln NB, Berman P. The effect of a stroke rehabilitation unit on functional and psychological outcome. A randomised controlled trial. *Cerebrovasc Dis* 1996;**6**:106–10.
9. Indredavik B, Bakke F, Solberg R *et al.* Benefit of stroke unit: a randomised controlled trial. *Stroke* 1991;**22**:1026–31.
10. Strand T, Asplund K, Eriksson S et al. A non-intensive stroke unit reduces functional disability and the need for long-term hospitalisation. *Stroke* 1985;**16**:29–34.
11. Kaste M, Palomaki H, Sarna S. Where and how should elderly stroke patients be treated? A randomized trial. *Stroke* 1995;**26**:249–53.
12. Aitken PD, Rodgers H, French JM, Bates D, James OFW. General medical or geriatric unit care for acute stroke? A controlled trial. *Age Ageing* 1993;**22** (suppl 2):4–5.
13. Kalra L, Eade J. Role of stroke rehabilitation units in managing severe disability after stroke. *Stroke* 1995;**26**:2031–4.
14. Stevens RS, Ambler NR, Warren MD. A randomised controlled trial of a stroke rehabilitation ward. *Age Ageing* 1984;**13**:65–75.

Chapter 6

1. Dennis M, Langhorne P. So stroke units save lives: where do we go from here? *Br Med J* 1994;**309**:1273–7.
2. Beech R, Ratcliffe M, Tilling K, Wolfe C, on behalf of the participants of the European Study of Stroke Care. Hospital services for stroke care. A European perspective. *Stroke* 1996;**27**:1958–64.
3. Wood-Dauphinee S, Shapiro S, Bass E. A randomised trial of team care following stroke. *Stroke* 1984;**5**:864–72.
4. Strand T, Asplund K, Eriksson S *et al.* A non-intensive stroke unit reduces functional disability and the need for long-term hospitalisation. *Stroke* 1985;**16**:29–34.
5. Hankey G, Deleo D, Stewart-Wynne EG. Acute hospital care for stroke patients: a randomised trial. *Cerebrovasc Dis* 1995;**5**:228.
6. Indredavik B, Bakke F, Solberg R *et al.* Benefit of stroke unit: a randomised controlled trial. *Stroke* 1991;**22**:1026–31.
7. Warlow CP, Dennis MS, van Gijn J *et al. Stroke: a practical guide to management.* Edinburgh: Blackwell Science, 1996.
8. International Stroke Trial Collaborative Group. The international stroke trial (IST): a randomised trial of aspirin, subcutaneous heparin, both, or neither among 19435 patients with acute ischaemic stroke. *Lancet* 1997;**349**:1569–81.
9. CAST (Chinese Acute Stroke Trial) Collaborative Group. CAST: randomised placebo-controlled trial of early aspirin use in 20000 patients with acute ischaemic stroke. *Lancet* 1997;**349**:1641–9.
10. Lincoln NB, Willis BA, Philips SA, Juby LC, Berman P. Comparison of rehabilitation practice on hospital wards for stroke patients. *Stroke* 1996;**27**:18–23.
11. Ashburn A, Partridge CJ, de Suza L. Physiotherapy and the rehabilitation of stroke: a review. *Clin Rehab* 1993;**7**:337–45.
12. Le Roux AA. TELFER: the concept. *Physiotherapy* 1993;**79**:755–8.
13. Wade D. Measurement in neurological rehabilitation. In: Wade D. Ed. *Activities of daily living (ADL) and extended ADL tests.* Oxford: Oxford University Press, 1990.

14. Wells PS, Lensing AWA, Hirsh J. Graduated compression stockings in the prevention of postoperative venous thromboembolism: a meta-analysis. *Ann Intern Med* 1994;**154**:67–72.
15. Forster A, Young J. Specialist nurse support for patients with stroke in the community: a randomised controlled trial. *Br Med J* 1996;**312**:1642–6.
16. Dennis M, O'Rourke S, Slattery J, Staniforth T, Warlow C. Evaluation of a stroke family care worker: results of a randomised controlled trial. *Br Med J* 1997;**314**:1071–6.
17. Stroke Unit Trialists' Collaboration. A collaborative systematic review of the randomised trials of organised inpatient (stroke unit) care after stroke. *Br Med J* 1997;**314**:1151–9.
18. Department of Health. *Health of the nation: a strategy for health in England.* London: HMSO, 1992.

Chapter 7

1. Gladman J, Barer D, Langhorne P. Specialist rehabilitation after stroke. Effective in the short term, but more work needed in the long term. *Br Med J* 1996;**312**:1623–4.
2. Wade DT, Langton-Hewer R, Skilbeck CE, Bainton D, Burns-Cox C. Controlled trial of a home-care service for acute stroke patients. *Lancet* 1985;**i**:323–6.
3. Warlow CP, Dennis MS, van Gijn J et al. *Stroke: a practical guide to management.* Edinburgh: Blackwell Science, 1996.
4. Young JB, Forster A. The Bradford community stroke trial: results at six months. *Br Med J* 1992;**304**:1085–9.
5. Gladman JRF, Lincoln NB, Barer DH. A randomised controlled trial of domiciliary and hospital-based rehabilitation for stroke patients after discharge from hospital. *J Neurol Neurosurg Psychiatr* 1993;**56**:960–6.
6. Gladman J, Forster A, Young J. Hospital- and home-based rehabilitation after discharge from hospital for stroke patients: analysis of two trials. *Age Ageing* 1995;**24**:49–53.
7. International Stroke Trial Collaborative Group. The international stroke trial (IST): a randomised trial of aspirin, subcutaneous heparin, both, or neither among 19435 patients with acute ischaemic stroke. *Lancet* 1997;**349**:1569–81.
8. CAST (Chinese Acute Stroke Trial) Collaborative Group. CAST: randomised placebo-controlled trial of early aspirin use in 20000 patients with acute ischaemic stroke. *Lancet* 1997;**349**:1641–9.

Appendix

1. Mays N, Pope C. *Qualitative research in health care.* London: BMJ Publishing Group, 1996.
2. Hankey G, Deleo D, Stewart-Wynne EG. Acute hospital care for stroke patients: a randomised trial. *Cerebrovasc Dis* 1995;**5**:228.
3. Indredavik B, Bakke F, Solberg R et al. Benefit of stroke unit: a randomised controlled trial. *Stroke* 1991;**22**:1026–31.
4. Kalra L, Dale P, Crome P. Improving stroke rehabilitation: a controlled study. *Stroke* 1993;**24**:1462–7.
5. Juby LC, Lincoln NB, Berman P. The effect of a stroke rehabilitation unit on functional and psychological outcome. A randomised controlled trial. *Cerebrovasc Dis* 1996;**6**:106–10.

Index